Harvesting Organs
&
Cherishing Life

What Christians Need to Know About Organ Donation and Procurement

Christopher W. Bogosh, RN-BC

Heidi Klessig, MD

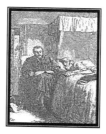

Good Samaritan Books

Foreword

Harvesting Organs & Cherishing Life is a necessary book. I found it enlightening, disturbing and occasionally infuriating. Having never written the Foreword to a book, I agreed to write this one because Christians must address the godless ethics behind organ donation and procurement. Furthermore, they must reject the modern definition of death, which has opened the door to greedy, scandalous, and even murderous practices in harvesting human organs. Please consider, then, the divinely orchestrated events that brought this book into existence.

The sovereign Lord, "who worketh all things after to the counsel of His own will" (Eph 1:11, KJV), included me in a remarkable chain of events. Mt. Zion Bible Church, the congregation I serve as a pastor, oversees Chapel Library (www.chapellibrary.org). This national and international literature ministry serves thousands of people in America and abroad. I am the General Editor of the *Free Grace Broadcaster* (FGB), a quarterly digest of Christ-centered sermons and articles.

In 2013, Robert Granger, a friend of Chapel Library, kindly gifted me with a book entitled *Compassionate Jesus: Rethinking the Christian's Approach to Modern Medicine* by Christopher W. Bogosh. I was unfamiliar with the author, but the title intrigued me. So, I mentally put the book into my sizable list of "books to read someday."

Compassionate Jesus would likely have suffered the doom of never arriving at "someday," but the opportunity surprisingly appeared in early 2020. As the editor of the FGB, I decided to address the subject of sickness. COVID-19 was everywhere. The virus was on everyone's minds and lips at the time. "Sickness," then, was the theme I chose for the next edition of the FGB. As I prayed about where to find biblical articles on sickness, *Compassionate Jesus* came to mind.

I plunged into Chris's book, and after the first chapter, I could not put it down. I was deeply moved and profoundly challenged by his biblical thoughts about medicine and healthcare. As I read chapter after chapter, I learned about the pagan notions behind our modern medical establishment. I also found myself repeatedly conscience-stricken as the book exposed my own unbiblical views about sickness and health. That was troubling—*painful.*

When a Christian, a pastor no less, discovers that something he believes has been more influenced by the unbelieving world than by God-breathed Scripture, heartfelt repentance is the only way ahead. So, there I found myself: enlightened, repentant, and humbled. The Word of God was correcting my erroneous thinking about medicine and healthcare.

That issue of the FGB was well-received, and not the least because of Chris's articles. That motivated me to do the next FGB on "Death and Dying." I discovered, to my surprise, that Joel Beeke and Chris had written a book together entitled *Dying and Death*! The book was so helpful that it was difficult to choose which chapters to use. Again, after prayer and much thought, I was convinced that Chris's treatment of brain death was something that all Christians needed to reckon with.

Chapel Library released the print version and the digital version of the FGB "Death and Dying" on August 25, 2020. Two days later, we received an email from Dr. Heidi Klessig. Her opening sentences were riveting: "Thank you for addressing 'brain death' in the latest *Free Grace Broadcaster*! This is a subject much neglected by the church and pro-life movement. As a result, families are ill-equipped and unprepared when a loved one becomes seriously ill, and medical 'experts' approach them with the proposal of considering 'brain dead' organ harvest." *Much neglected by the church and pro-life movement* (italics mine) – troubling words!

Dr. Klessig's closing paragraph was equally gripping: "I understand that in God's providence, decisions to harvest organs have been made, often in ignorance of the facts. God is merciful, and so should we be as His Body. I have a great dread of being 'controversial' or of burdening people with unbiblical burdens. However, as I was once the anesthesiologist who turned off the ventilator on these vulnerable patients, I now want to be part of the solution in bringing these issues to light for the church." Heidi's words moved me!

I knew that Chris would be encouraged by Dr. Klessig's email and immediately forwarded it to him. The next thing I knew, Chris copied me on an email to her, inviting her to write a book with him about brain death and organ harvesting. He closed that correspondence with these words: "I have to say, it was through a remarkable web of God's providences that we have come into contact." That remarkable web of God's providences is why this book is in print and why I am writing its Foreword!

The authors of *Harvesting Organs & Cherishing Life* do not oppose organ donation and transplants; instead, they propose a view that does not violate the Law of God. Their abundant and verifiable examples of the dark side of organ harvesting will be repulsive, even horrifying to some. Their explanation of human death not only corrects the modern brain death error but exalts the victory of Jesus Christ over death. The biblical arguments *will* provoke readers: some will agree, some will disagree. But by God's grace, many will repent and renounce the godless ethics of organ harvesting. I know, for I am thankfully in the third group.

While one may not agree with every argument offered or every conclusion the authors draw from Scripture, they have done their homework. The unlawful taking of human life is a direct assault on God Himself, for He created man in His image. God decreed before He created the universe to send His eternal Son into this sinful world to die an actual death — death in total with all its horror, not brain death. Christ's death conquers death. By dying on the cross of Golgotha, Jesus paid the penalty for the sins of God's people. And when He rose from the dead three days later, He conquered death forever.

But brain death is man's creation, often used to serve his greed in organ harvesting. Those who stand for the beauty of God-created life against abortion and euthanasia need to hear the alarm this book sounds. More, they need to raise their voices against murdering still-living human beings for their organs and exalt Christ's triumph over death (Rom 6:23).

You cannot read this book and remain indifferent to the authors' arguments. From a friend's gift to publishing this book, God's sovereign hand has put *Harvesting Organs & Cherishing Life* in *your* hands. And you are now entering the realm of controversy. Although Dr. Klessig dreads being controversial, she and Chris will not escape it with this book! But they have raised their voices in this controversy with grace, mercy, love, and holy boldness, holding forth the words of life in Jesus Christ the Lord.

To the God of life be all the glory!

Pastor Jeff Pollard
Mt. Zion Bible Church
Pensacola, FL

Preface

Harvesting Organs & Cherishing Life: What Christians Need to Know About Organ Donation and Procurement was brought to life by the Creator of life, who gave us life at conception and the inspiration in middle life to write it! As noted in the Foreword by Pastor Pollard, a remarkable set of providences converged to give birth to this book. We have a debt of gratitude to offer each of the lives involved in this project, but first, a few comments to prepare the living, heart beating, and breathing reader.

This book may not be an easy read for some Christians. We reveal shocking facts about modern organ procurement practices occurring in America and the world today, and our book's two-fold position is direct, uncompromising, and absolute: (1) image-bearers of God (human beings) have worth no matter what condition they are in, and (2) human beings are still alive when biological signs of life exist in their bodies. Thus, ending the life of these people is murder in God's eyes. We believe this position to be empirical, straightforward, and biblical.

Harvesting Organs & Cherishing Life does not oppose transplanting organs and tissues. Donating blood, a kidney, or even a whole biologically dead body are excellent acts of self-giving, provided no one is exploited or forced. Our book draws the line at manipulative actions that are harmful to others and dishonor the living God, who gives the spirit of life to people.

The Nazi "life unworthy of life" (*Lebensunwertes Leben*) eugenics program comes to mind regarding the modern organ harvest agenda. Forced organ harvesting from Uighurs at concentration camps in China is a present reality, an atrocity the Biden administration ignores. In the United States (US), we use phrases like "quality of life" to assign value to human life. This phrase is really nothing more than a dressed-up version of the Nazi doctrine "life unworthy of life."

Some people against abortion, but in favor of modern organ harvesting, view in-utero cells as a "life in potential" to distinguish them from a fully developed "brain dead" donor with a beating heart and life story. Proponents of this idea see the latter possesses a "life unworthy of life" because of a *presumed* loss of potential. In the minds of those supporting the abominable *Lebensunwertes Leben*, those dubbed the *Untermensch* (sub-humans) should "Give the Gift of Life"—*literally*—to those judged more worthy of living.

The modern organ harvest business is immoral and unethical, and Christians need to oppose it (Matt. 6:13). In *Harvesting Organs & Cherishing Life,* we set naturalism in the context of a Christian worldview. Biology proves that life begins at conception and does not end until cellular processes switch from functions that promote life to death, decay, and recycling the body. As the Bible teaches, "the body without the spirit is dead" (James 2:26, KJV). Natural life ends sometime after cardiopulmonary function ceases—this is the science—any other definition of death is based on a worldview.

This is our journey as Christians and healthcare professionals with numerous years of experience. We believe *all* Christians need to hear our message and consider it. Therefore, our goal was to make this book as accessible as possible. We've intentionally written in a clear and engaging style, without footnotes, endnotes, or academic concerns in mind. We merely cite our research in the book's body, and nothing in *Harvesting Organs & Cherishing Life* is obscure.

In fact, one of the biggest surprises was how available the material we wrote about was. Numerous online newspaper and magazine articles mention the modern human body-part harvesting business and its questionable ethics. Investigative journalists have aired programs, and physicians have written books about today's legal definition of death and organ procurement practices. Congressional hearings have also taken place due to injustices related to all these matters. If the reader wants to confirm our sources, an internet search is all that's needed.

Now a brief word to acknowledge those who helped us with *Harvesting Organs & Cherishing Life*. Foremost, a special thanks to Pastor Jeff Pollard for bringing us together. If Jeff did not write about modern medicine's definition of death in the *Free Grace Broadcaster*, we would've never come into contact with each other. Of course, we are convinced that these events were not random, including our exposure to the pioneering work of Dr. Ed Payne. Doctor Payne's dedication to promoting a biblical worldview for medical science helped both of us in our professions, and not the least, to write a book as bold as this!

We would like to thank Natalya Bartelt for creating the book cover. We could not ask for a better jacket to reflect the contents of *Harvesting Organs & Cherishing Life*. The team of proofreaders offered honest, essential, and critical feedback. Thank you, Melissa Gaitley, Gail Yule, Brent Evans, and Pastor Chris Ames. The book was made more explicit due to your intervention. Of course, a special thanks to our brothers and sisters in Christ, whose unceasing prayers and fellowship brought strength to our "feeble arms and weak knees" (Isa. 35:3).

Last but certainly not least, we would like to thank our spouses, Robin and Darrel. I suppose an entire book could be written about their support as proofreaders, encouragers, and devoted partners. Although *Harvesting Organs & Cherishing Life* is not a large book, the amount of time and effort invested in research and writing was still significant. This placed an enormous burden on our spouses, so thank you for living out Galatians 6:2.

Finally, a word to acknowledge those mentioned in this book, especially Heather and Hannah. Their experience displays the best of organ transplant medicine. We are thankful for their willingness to share their intimate testimony. For the rest, well read on. When doing so, please remember that God breathes life into human beings at conception. He cherishes the life he gives to this person until the heart, lungs, and brain—all three—cease to function and the God-breathed spirit separates from the body.

Christopher W. Bogosh, RN-BC
Heidi Klessig, MD

Contents

Abbreviations

Computer Tomography (CT)

Dead Donor Rule (DDR)

Donors after Circulatory Death (DCD)

Electroencephalogram (EEG)

Intensive Care Unit (ICU)

Intravenous (IV)

Magnetic Resonance Imaging (MRI)

Minimally Conscious State (MCS)

Near Death Experience (NDE)

Operating Room (OR)

Organ Procurement Organization (OPO)

Organ Transplantation Network (OPTN)

Out of Body Experience (OBE)

Patient Self Determination Act (PSDA)

Persistent Vegetative State (PVS)

Physician Assisted Suicide (PAS)

Return of Spontaneous Circulation (ROSC)

Uniform Anatomical Gift Act (UAGA)

Uniform Determination of Death Act (UDDA)

United Network for Organ Sharing (UNOS)

United States (US)

World Health Organization (WHO)

Introduction:
Death in the ICU and Organ Donors

Of all the topics Christians would like to study, death in an intensive care unit (ICU) is probably not one of them. You may be thinking, "What does this have to do with *Harvesting Organs & Cherishing Life*?" Aside from a selfless living organ donor and a blessed recipient who continue to live after an organ transplant, everything. In the ICU, the organ donor permission on a person's driver's license, perhaps your own, becomes a legal *mandate* under the Uniform Anatomical Gift Act (UAGA) to donate body parts in most states. Maybe you were not aware of this.

For example, John Flath, age 18, died in 2011 after a workout with Army Reserve Officer Training Corp (ROTC) cadets. John was a healthy teenager, who excelled at sports, had a promising future, and a family who loved him.

Since his cause of death was not known, John's parents wanted to find out why he died. Sadly, due to the UAGA and John's registration as an organ donor, they could not.

In fact, the UAGA mandate has upended criminal investigations across the United States (US). The *Los Angeles Times* and *Chicago Tribune* reported on this pervasive problem. Believe it or not, organ procurement organizations (OPOs) swoop in on the recently deceased like hungry vultures to pick apart bodies before forensic specialists can examine them! As a result, the causes of death cannot be determined due to aggressive body-part collecting practices that are protected by the UAGA, and clues cannot be gathered to arrest violent criminals.

Another shocking truth you may not know about is that many organ donors declared dead by US law are still alive. The Uniform Determination of Death Act (UDDA) and Dead Donor Rule (DDR) are legal fictions. They are not valid according to the biological facts of life. Like abortion, this legislation permits a brutal act upon a defenseless human with God's breath of life. It is not the episode that landed most organ donors in the ICU that causes natural death but the organ removal process itself.

The UDDA defines death in two ways: "(1) irreversible cessation of circulatory and respiratory functions, or (2) irreversible cessation of all functions of the entire brain, including the brainstem, is dead." This definition sounds careful, but it is seriously flawed, as the reader will see in chapter three. Not the least is separating the brain from the heart and lungs; the impossible standard of "irreversible cessation" that is never actually met; and ultimately its biased and subjective application in clinical practice to allow organ harvesting under the DDR.

More than ninety percent of the organ donors in ICUs are declared "brain dead," and they still have beating hearts. The rest, donors after cardiac or circulatory death (DCD), still have brain activity, but their heart needs assistance to beat. During the operation to remove their organs, both require anesthesia like any other person undergoing surgery. Not only does the anesthesia reduce the suffering in a donor that's defined dead, but the donor's response to the anesthetics proves he or she is still alive.

Aside from these horrible truths, pro-life people profess belief in life beginning at conception, which is several weeks before a heart, lungs, brain, and conscious experience develop. This raises the question, "Why do Christians denounce abortion but condone organ donation and procurement under the UDDA and DDR?" Christians must grapple with these issues if they want to be consistent, pro-life, and, most importantly, faithful to Holy Scripture.

We anticipate a whole range of emotions at this point—disbelief, anger, guilt—but please don't put down *Harvesting Organs & Cherishing Life: What Christians Need to Know About Organ Donation and Procurement*. What is written in this book is essential to understand. It presents clear scientific facts about natural life and death, biblical guidance to honor the living God, encouragement for those stricken with remorse, and horrific truths about organ procurement practices worldwide, including right here in America.

What follows is not from two armchair academics. It is from a Christian doctor and nurse with nearly a half-century of combined medical experience. We've cared for hundreds of people in critical conditions. Both of us also entered our careers after death was redefined by the UDDA in 1981. We know the laws, ethical dilemmas, medical hubris, and the ICU. We also know signs of life and biological death.

Aside from conditions like congestive heart failure (CHF), chronic obstructive pulmonary disease (COPD), birth issues, and post-operative recovery, a person often ends up in the ICU after a traumatic event. The emergency medical service (EMS) responds to a 911 call, arrives on the scene, initiates life support, and transports the person to the hospital for life-saving care. In most cases, this individual cannot respond to the environment. He or she is entirely dependent on doctors, nurses, and family members to survive.

When the person arrives at the emergency department (ED), a breathing tube has been inserted in the mouth that directs air to the lungs (intubated). The heart may have been shocked to restart it (defibrillated), or it may be stimulated by large pads on the chest and back to cause it to beat (paced). The person will have intravenous (IV) medications flowing into the body and any bodily injuries stabilized. Eventually, the critically ill person is transferred to the ICU.

In the ICU, the non-responsive individual will be hooked up to a dizzying array of wires attached to pads outside the body and lines entering it. Numerous beeps and alarms will be heard. The breathing tube is now attached to a ventilator with its own sounds, most notably air going in and out (inspiration and expiration). Treatment stabilizes vital signs (blood pressure, heart rate, respiratory rate, oxygen levels, and temperature), reduces swelling, corrects traumatic injuries, and addresses infections.

Aside from analyzing numerous blood samples, x-rays, and other ultrasounds and scans, the non-responsive person will be assessed frequently with the Glasgow Coma Scale (GCS). This bedside exam evaluates neurological function, and the score ranges from three (non-responsive) to fifteen (responsive). As time passes, formal testing to declare brain death will start if a cardiac arrest and biological death do not occur. We will consider this testing in chapter three.

Once brain death is determined, treatment in the ICU shifts to preserving body parts for registered and potential organ donors. Maybe you were not aware of this either. Later in the book, we will consider the tragic case of Jahi McMath, a thirteen-year-old girl declared legally dead by UDDA criteria in California. Her mother did not consent to donate her organs, so a withdrawal of medical care, nutrition, and hydration occurred against her mother's wishes. According to US law, Jahi had a "life unworthy of life." She lived for five more years in New Jersey.

I (Chris) recently watched *Roe vs. Wade* (2021), an off shoot of *The Silent Scream* from 1984. The movie was a gruesome portrayal of the abortion movement in the 1970s, along with its political corruption, greed, and manipulative tactics. The narrator of the film, Dr. Bernard N. Nathanson, was once an arrogant obstetrician who converted from pro-choice to pro-life.

By Nathanson's own admission, he was obsessed with murdering the unborn. He did so under the guise of doing good for others. His goal was to provide pregnant women with a safe abortion and the hope for a better future without the burden of a child. Later in life, he realized the evil of the pro-choice delusion he was dedicated to following, as well as his hatred toward the Creator of life.

Just like *Roe vs. Wade* allowed the murder of an unconscious baby, the UDDA and DDR permit the murder of non-responsive people with signs of life. Both permissions have nothing to do with facts or science but everything to do with a philosophical understanding of human nature and a worldview. Holy Scripture and traditional Christianity has a great deal to say about these issues, along with living out the Christian faith in a country that manipulates the truth, devalues life, and cancels anyone who opposes secular morals.

While this book focuses on the aggressive organ procurement agenda in the US, there is a dark side to this business worldwide. We already mentioned the forced organ harvesting in

China, but other exploitative practices are occurring globally. We will present some of these matters in chapter two. Since these are human rights issues and crimes against humanity, they have come on the radar of Christians and non-Christians alike. Nevertheless, using legal fictions to declare organ donors dead and harvesting their body parts, while they still have biological signs of life, is a tragedy Christians in America need to confront!

The transplant business has told numerous lies, deceptions some honest healthcare professionals are questioning today. Christians need to hear the truth about organ harvesting practices that start in the ICU after a death declaration under the UDDA and those occurring worldwide. Nevertheless, all is not a loss with organ donation and transplants. Christians can still engage in this medical blessing in wise and selfless ways, provided they honor God and cherish life. We will consider one in the next chapter.

1

Donating a Kidney

Hannah is a young woman in her thirties born with a genetic disorder that causes kidney failure. At age twelve, she needed a kidney transplant. Dialysis, the process of filtering the blood by a machine, would've helped Hannah for a while. Still, Hannah's inevitable outcome at this young age without a new kidney was death.

After Hannah was diagnosed, the entire family rallied to her side. Everyone wanted to give her a kidney, but there were a few more obstacles to navigate. First, Hannah needed a kidney from a matching donor. Second, she and the donor required an organ transplant surgery that was not cheap. Third, Hannah would need to take antirejection drugs for the rest of her life, and these medications are expensive. By the grace of God, all these obstacles were overcome. Hannah's mother, Heather, was Hannah's best match for a kidney, and Heather was more than willing to give it.

Hannah's body thrived in her mother's womb for nine months, and now Heather would sustain Hannah's body for the rest of her life. When I (Heidi) asked Heather about how she felt, "I was scared," she said, "but I knew I had to do this to save my daughter's life." As a result of this surgery and the unique struggles they shared, the mother and daughter have a relational bond that is even more intimate. A union medical science helped to create.

Heather recalled the kind treatment of the medical staff during the transplant surgery. "We were wheeled to the operating room together. After my kidney was removed, I remember being told that it would be hand-carried to the operating room where Hannah was waiting to receive it. I just loved thinking of that!" A quick and careful transfer of a perfused organ is an outright necessity to ensure a successful organ transplant.

Having transplant surgery is relatively easy, thanks to anesthesia, but recovery is difficult, especially if complications occur, which they did. Heather opened her worn Bible with underlined verses, and with watery eyes, pointed to Romans 8:35 and read aloud: "Who shall separate us from the love of Christ? Shall trouble or hardship or persecution or famine or nakedness or danger or sword?" Then she slid her finger to verse 37, "No," with a bold tone in her voice, "in all these things we are more than conquerors through him who loved us!" Looking into my eyes, Heather said, "this was our hope in recovery and pulled us through the difficulties."

After the post-surgical recovery was completed, they were able to return home. Both faced challenges and celebrated victories. "It was a difficult year," Heather recounted. More than twenty years have passed since the transplant. Still, medical monitoring, laboratory testing, and medications have continued, especially for Hannah.

Thanks to Heather, Hannah is now part of a pioneering generation of survivors. She was one of the few who survived her childhood disease at the time. Even though her kidney function has improved, she still has health problems due to her genetic disorder. Yet, amid her adversity, Hannah devoted her life to Jesus, pursued an advanced degree, and overcame horrendous obstacles. She is an inspiration to young women and an advocate for the disability community.

Hannah and Heather's story is a beautiful testimony of a mother's love for her daughter and advances in medical science. It is also an inspiring story of giving even one's organ to benefit another person.

Registered Organ Donors and the UDDA

While donating a kidney is the most frequent living donor gift, other organs and tissues may be given. Of course, blood comes to mind, which started in the 18th century and was dramatically refined during World War II. Living donors can also donate a portion of their liver, skin, bone marrow, and stem cells. Make no mistake, however. Donating organs and tissues as a willing donor who will continue to live is different from being a *registered* organ donor under the Uniform Determination of Death Act (UDDA).

Having an organ donor card or designation on a driver's license is an act of civic duty that is potentially suicidal because of the UDDA. Anyone over eighteen can become an organ donor. In fact, about fifty-eight percent of the people in the United States (US) made this snap decision at Department of Motor Vehicle (DMV) sites around the nation! A choice influenced by eager advertisements with deceptive tactics.

The US has an aggressive organ recruitment propaganda program. February 14 is designated National Organ Donation Day, and organ procurement organizations (OPOs) serve as organ advocates in America. For the Christian, however, all this nationalist pride is misguided because of the redefining of death in 1981.

Doctor Henry Beecher wrote an article in the *Journal of the American Medical Association* with the classic title: "A Definition of Irreversible Coma: Report of the Ad Hoc Committee of the

Harvard Medical School to Examine the Definition of Brain Death." This article, written in 1968, laid the foundation for the UDDA in 1981.

What was the driving force behind Beecher's article? "Our primary purpose is to define irreversible coma as a new criterion for death," writes Beecher. He continues, "There are two reasons why there is need for a definition:

(1) improvements in resuscitative and supportive measures have led to increased efforts to save those who are desperately injured. Sometimes these efforts have only a partial success so that the result is an individual whose heart continues to beat but whose brain is irreversibly damaged. The burden is great on patients who suffer permanent loss of intellect, on their families, on the hospitals, and on those in need of hospital beds already occupied by these comatose patients.

(2) Obsolete criteria for the definition of death can lead to controversy in obtaining organs for transplantation."

Beecher wanted to eliminate those who were a burden to society and help those more fortunate. Sounds like the Nazi "life unworthy of life" doctrine. Those with a *supposed* "permanent loss of intellect" with beating hearts are an annoyance to themselves, their families, medical institutions, and the more privileged "in need of hospital beds."

In Beecher's mind, however, these newly defined "brain dead" sub-humans or "cadavers" in a *presumed* "irreversible coma" are not entirely useless. Society can make use of them as organ donors. If labeled legally dead while still alive on life support, their perfused body parts can be harvested and transplanted into those regarded as more worthy of living.

The UDDA is a social policy at odds with the worldview of Holy Scripture. The sixth commandment is clear, "You shall not murder" (Exo. 20:13). It is the revealed will of God for people not to murder themselves (suicide), others (homicide), or to be complicit in the act of murder. The sixth commandment, not the UDDA, lays the moral foundation and ethical parameters for Christian behavior.

Further, the Bible is also explicit about the

beginning of life, how we are to cherish it, and when natural death occurs. We will consider these issues in greater depth in chapter four. For now, however, it's important to note three biblical points: (1) life begins at conception, (2) human life has value because it reflects God's image, and (3) natural death occurs sometime after cardiopulmonary activity stops. Holy Scripture is clear about these matters.

Since it's against the will of God to choose an abortion or physician-assisted suicide (PAS), it can't be in line with God's will to register as an organ donor. Legally dead organ donors have biological signs of life, so they are not dead according to a biblical or empirical standard for death under the UDDA. To designate oneself as a *registered* organ donor is an act of self-sacrifice to a nation with a Nazi-like agenda, not devotion to God's will as revealed in Holy Scripture (see Acts 5:29).

The Effects of the Anonymous Donor Policy

After the first successful kidney transplants, physicians believed that introducing recipients to donors would improve clinical outcomes and establish a relationship forged by intimacy and gratitude. Like Hannah and Heather, a unique bond would develop. Nevertheless, the anonymous organ donor policy forbids this relationship, and travesties of injustice have followed as a result.

On May 18, 2021, Frank Fang of *Epoch Times* wrote: "Organ Donation Worker Exposes China's Money-Driven Transplant Industry." Fang interviewed a former organ procurement coordinator. According to the article, the representative was motivated to speak out against China's corrupt organ harvesting practices. The person did so at significant risk.

The individual reported that Chinese organ procurement organizations (OPOs) offer bribes to families to donate organs from vulnerable household members. According to the person interviewed, organ donation coordinators target poor people, and they do so with the help of doctors and police officers, who receive kickbacks. The poverty-stricken receive a promise of paid medical bills, a financial reward, and a pat on the back for "devotion to a greater good."

According to Fang's article, the family will receive a commission after consent to harvest is obtained. The coordinator mentioned the sad case where a donor could have lived on with non-aggressive medical treatment. Instead, the family decided to donate the organs of the loved one for a price. The article also mentions family members who were alive but mentally impaired, whose organs were sold.

Exploiting the vulnerable for profit is a travesty of justice, but there is even a darker side to China's practices the American anonymous donor policy helps to protect. In 2016, Dr. Thomas Diflo, a kidney doctor at New York University's Medical Center, was called to testify before Congress. Former dialysis patients of his received kidney transplants without his knowledge. The recipients returned to Diflo for follow-up care.

When Diflo asked where the kidneys came from, some said from unknown donors in China. Investigators discovered they may not have just come from exploited poor people. They were more likely from political prisoners executed expressly for the purpose of harvesting and selling their organs!

Thankfully, Texas lawmakers recently passed legislation to expose and condemn China's egregious practices. The April 23, 2021 article in *Epoch News*, "Texas Senate Passes Resolution to Curb China's Forced Organ Harvesting: 'There Needs to Be a Global Outcry,'" explains the legislation. The article also featured a picture of Asians marching in the streets of New York with signs: "China: Stop Murdering for Organs."

When the supply chain is shrouded in darkness, abuses will follow. The anonymous donor tenet in the US has also promoted "transplant tourism." Since 2006, this practice has skyrocketed. In 2021, Canada made transplant tourism a crime, but it is still legal in America. Statistics from the World Health Organization (WHO) indicate a transplant tourist can pay between $70,000 to $160,000 depending on the organ involved. Those US citizens who received kidneys from unknown donors in China paid a mere $10,000!

The veil of secrecy promotes this venture—

an anonymous supply chain of organs from paid, forced, or altruistic donors worldwide and right here in the US. A few years ago, I (Chris) watched an earnest pastor end his sermon in tears. He fell to his knees in front of the congregation and cried out with clasped hands, "stop murdering unborn babies!"

A few weeks later, the same pastor invited a frail and pale-looking man wearing a respiratory mask to the pulpit to give a testimony. Recently, he had heart-lung transplant surgery from an anonymous donor, who was declared dead under the UDDA. The grateful recipient concluded in a soft voice: "I don't know who the donor was, but I am grateful to have his organs."

What if he met the donor in the intensive care unit (ICU)? What if he saw the beating heart on a monitor and heard the lungs aerating? What if he received a layman's explanation describing why this donor with a beating heart was declared "dead" and the non-donor on life support in the same condition was not? What if he looked at the potential costs for his one transplant surgery? All of this, obscured—why? Is it to protect the donor's anonymity or hide ugly truths about America's organ procurement business?

One of the strategies employed by pro-life groups is to offer ultrasounds for women contemplating abortion. The goal is to show the mother the developing baby in the womb is alive. Technicians point out the beating heart and describe the growing body. Pro-choice groups object to this tactic, just like pro-harvest groups oppose full transparency. The donor mentioned above is a fully developed person with a beating heart and life story. Only the wicked, confused, or afraid would end a baby's life attached to a placenta or remove organs from a heart-beating person connected to life support.

We have come a long way from a loving mother donating a kidney to her daughter selflessly and transparently in an intimate way. Today, all types of tissues and organs are harvested from unnamed donors declared dead under the legal fiction of the UDDA. As a result of the American anonymous donor policy, injustices occur worldwide and right here in the US.

Presently, we are in a realm where death has been redefined. Deceptive tactics to obtain organs are employed. Vulnerable people are exploited, and a lucrative human body-part market has emerged.

2

The Organ Procurement Business

The United Network for Organ Sharing (UNOS) regulates the allocation of organs and tissues in America. Intricately connected with UNOS are fifty-eight non-profit organ procurement organizations (OPOs) located strategically throughout the United States (US). These groups are under the Organ Procurement and Transplantation Network (OPTN).

According to UNOS's most recent 2021 statistics, about 108,100 people are on the US national waiting list for an organ. In 2020, 39,035 organ transplants were performed in America. Due to a lack of organs, roughly seventeen people die every day. The demand for organs significantly outnumbers the supply by 69,065. On average, there is a five-year wait time to receive an organ transplant.

This is the narrative transplant surgeons, hospitals, and pharmaceutical companies want Americans to focus on, but it's not without untoward consequences. When the focus is on the scarcity of organs and a promise of a miraculous rebirth after receiving a new one, unscrupulous acts motivated by greed and need are bound to follow. Physicians, OPOs, and medical institutions control the organ transplant message and standards. They are also responsible for increasing the donor pool.

Since the first kidney transplant in 1954 and heart transplant in 1967, a few attempts were made to increase America's donor pool. The first move was in 1968 with the Uniform Anatomical Gift Act (UAGA). Intricately connected to the UAGA was a push to create brain-death criteria, codified as law in 1981 as the Uniform Determination of Death Act (UDDA). The UAGA permitted organ donation. The UDDA redefined death to authorize the harvesting of perfused organs from unresponsive people on life support with hearts still pulsating in their chests.

Another attempt to expand the pool of donors came in revisions to the UAGA, first in 1987 and later in 2006. The 2006 revision made a registered donor's desire to donate supersede his or her same rights under the Patient Self Determination Act (PSDA) of 1997. Under this regulation, life-support to preserve organs and tissues will continue regardless of prior instructions to withdraw it.

Even if a legally appointed family member or surrogate attempts to enforce these advance directives, the UAGA trumps that right. Aggressive medical treatment with the intent to keep the body alive, under the delusion the donor is dead, will continue! The 2006 UAGA reform requires the treating doctor to notify the regional OPO and to begin the harvest process. A person's desire to be a registered organ donor is now a *mandate* to donate in most states, regardless of prior directives protected by the PSDA.

Even with these attempts to increase the donor pool, the demand still exceeds the supply more than double today. Scott Carney, *The Red Market*, writes: "Transplant lists like the one perpetually updated by the United Network for Organ Sharing bloat as doctors tell dying patients that the only way to save their lives is to receive a functioning liver or kidney to replace the failing parts in their own bodies." This message creates a crisis for someone with a failing organ and a problem well-meaning people want to fix.

Considering this dilemma, some in the US advocate mandatory organ donation for all legally dead people on life-support. Others, who are less radical, suggest that people opt out of donating organs on a driver's license or another legal instrument rather than opt-in. This practice occurs in the United Kingdom (UK). Some in America believe red markets (selling body parts for a profit) are the answer.

Selling Body Parts: The Red Market

A red market may sound like a feasible solution in a country driven by capitalism, even for some Christians. A person may think, "Why not sell a kidney to someone in need? If it's legitimate to donate one for free, why not receive a monetary gift in the process? After all, it's my body." This practice occurs in Iran and other parts of the world, but it's laden with problems. We will consider these issues later. From a biblical perspective, however, selling organs, tissues, and body fluids (e.g., bone marrow, blood products, eggs, and sperm) is immoral and unethical.

Holy Scripture has a lot to say about selling oneself to a stranger, as a prostitute sells him- or herself, and about giving oneself, such as two people in marriage (cf. 1 Cor. 6:15–20). In both situations, people share their bodies with other people. The latter is a selfless act of giving to a known person intimately (like Heather donating a kidney to Hannah); the former sells his or her body "part" to a stranger for a profit. There is no selflessness, self-giving, and intimacy in selling one's body, even in parts.

This does not mean a great deal of pimping and profit making are not occurring in the US! Like an elaborate prostitution ring, local OPOs collect body parts from altruistic donors, OPTN manages them, and UNOS allocates them. One cornea (a part of the eye) as a replacement is worth $3,150. A single small piece of a rib ground up for a nose job, $510. The ulna forearm bone for a replacement $3,400. Ground bone mixed with stem cells for back surgeries, $2,550 for one teaspoon. After harvesting and processing fees are added, these body parts are sold to medical institutions.

Doctors, hospitals, and pharmaceutical companies rake in billions by implanting organs and tissues in people's bodies, and by ensuring they continue to function. For example, according to the 2020 Milliman Research Report: a kidney transplant surgery costs about $442,500, a heart transplant surgery $1,664,800, and a bone marrow tissue transplant procedure $1,071,700 in America. These profits do not include the income for procedures to prepare for the transplant surgeries, medications, and for a lifetime of follow-up care until the person dies.

The demand for transplantable organs and tissues has created a worldwide red market. The red market sells human goods, such as organs, tissues, bones, body fluids, and even whole bodies. In January of 2009, *Newsweek* published "Organ Trafficking is No Myth," and the article revealed that red market transactions occur in the US. The red market is a middleman supply business that appeases the human commodities demand, like the situation mentioned above.

For organs, by far, the item coveted most is kidneys. *The Guardian* reported in 2012 that kidney transactions were seventy-five percent of the red market business. In 2007, transplant tourists accounted for two-thirds of Pakistan's commercial organ market, in which 2,500 kidneys were sold that year. Kidney reimbursement can range from hundreds to thousands of dollars, depending on who the donor is, what the recipient is willing to pay, and the greed of those involved in the transaction.

IndUShealth and UnitedHealth Group provide options for their members to travel outside the US to receive kidney transplants. These companies have contacts with medical institutions in India, Pakistan, and Egypt. The transplant prices outside America are a lot less, and a network is set up for these kidney sales. Even though the World Health Organization (WHO) condemns the practice, it's still legal in the US. In 2006, the lower transplant costs motivated the West Virginia legislature to consider a formal out-of-country plan for state employees.

Aside from the corrupt organ business in China, Iran is the only country that permits above-board legal compensation for kidney donors. The practice was initially allowed in the 1980s, and it is only open to Iranian citizens, but like China, injustices abound. Under this program, the donor receives a tax credit, free health care, and a payment of $1,200 from the recipient for the kidney. The program, however, exploits Iranian citizens.

Over seventy percent of Iranian kidney donors are poverty-stricken. Due to economic setbacks, many see it as a solution to provide for their families. They never get the lift out of poverty they had hoped, however, and the same is true for those who sell kidneys in India, Egypt, and Pakistan.

As for paid donors outside Iran, many receive a small sum before the harvest surgery, but the organ broker disappears after the kidney is removed. Financial gains are short-lived for these exploited people. Due to adverse physical and mental outcomes after the surgery, most become disabled and unable to work. Nevertheless, the transplant tourist goes on with life satisfied with the bloody bargain, blissfully ignorant of the hardship of the anonymous donor.

Taking Organs: The Black Market

Aside from the questionable red market, a worldwide black market plagues the world. This includes a complex network of donors, third-party brokers, recipients, physicians, and hospitals. The cruelest participants in this business are organized crime syndicates and oppressive regimes that steal organs by forcing healthy adults, teenagers, and children to give them up.

As noted in the last chapter, this black market had connections to America. In 2016 the US House of Representatives held a hearing to investigate. The committee published *Organ Harvesting: An Examination of a Brutal Practice*. Dr. Diflo was called to testify before Congress and others. The House confirmed the forced organ harvesting occurring worldwide with connections to America. Still, as noted in the *Epoch News* article mentioned earlier, real federal action has been minimal.

China is well-known for removing organs from subjugated people. In 1978, a political prisoner was executed for a kidney, and in 1984 a law was passed that permitted the use of "deceased" prisoner's bodies by the Chinese Communist Party (CCP). During the 1990s, it was reported that political prisoners were used as organ donors.

Doctors Against Forced Organ Harvesting met a Chinese doctor and interviewed him about China's transplant policies. The physician reported that he was obligated by the CCP to procure political prisoners' livers and kidneys. The prisoners were summarily executed, and their organs were harvested because they disagreed with CCP policies.

In 1999, the CCP arrested and imprisoned Mandarin Chinese, who were Falun Gong practitioners. The devotees of this religion are about ten percent of the Chinese population. After the group was officially condemned, the regime forced them to submit to blood and tissue typing. Then the prisoners were placed on an organ donor list. It is estimated that 1.5 million Falun Gong were murdered by having their organs harvested.

David Matas and David Kilgour, who also testified before Congress in 2016, reported the Falun Gong account in *Bloody Harvest*. In 2014, Ethan Gutman published *The Slaughter,* which details the same atrocities. In 2016, both books' authors moved beyond Falun Gong's forced harvesting to expose organ procurement from the Uighurs, Tibetans, and Christians. In China today, it is estimated one or two million Uighur Muslims and other dissident groups are interred at CCP concentration camps in China's Xinjiang province.

According to a US national security specialist Brian T. Kennedy, "the government harvests the organs." It sells them "both in China and abroad." He continues: "This latter atrocity has become a multi-billion-dollar industry: the Uighur organs, since they are uncorrupted by alcohol or pork, are especially desirable to wealthy Muslims in the Middle East and elsewhere." Although China denies these allegations, the facts speak for themselves, and many Americans are complicit.

Doctors Against Forced Organ Harvesting reported that the practice of compelled harvesting continues in China today. It is a tremendous boon to its economy. Americans travel to China for organ transplants, and US insurance companies like UnitedHealth Group will even pay for these surgeries. China's challenge is not the lack of organs to transplant or immunosuppressant medications (another boost to the Chinese economy). It is the shortage of qualified medical personnel to perform transplants.

Once again, America fills this void by training Chinese doctors. The CCP will pay US universities to educate medical students. While attending a church in Cambridge, Massachusetts, I (Chris) met several students at Harvard University, Massachusetts Institute of Technology, and Boston University on scholarships funded by foreign governments. American institutions train many of these doctors on how to perform transplant surgeries. Those who receive CCP funding are expected to return to China to practice medicine.

Making Organs: Frankensteinish Greed

In August of 2015, pro-life people were horrified by the red market fetal body part dealings of Planned Parenthood (PP). A group disguised as the Center for Medical Progress posed as organ brokers. The undercover agents met with high-ranking officials from PP and secretly filmed the encounters. Hours of digital footage were posted on YouTube.

Deborah Nucatola, senior director of medical research at PP, quipped, "I'd say a lot of people want a liver . . . intact hearts . . . We've been very good at getting heart, lung, liver." These aborted babies have developing organs, bones, and tissues with specialized cells in a state of growth, so they are valuable to harvest.

In PP's eyes, the unborn baby is an attachment to the mother's body, just like a non-responsive heart-beating donor is attached to life support. After the woman exercised her "reproductive rights" to abort her fetus, why not harvest the remains? After all, this is what OPOs and medical institutions are doing with other people's organs, bones, and tissues.

Michele Goodwin, *Black Markets: The Supply and Demand of Human Body Parts*, wrote about the incident. In her "Planned Parenthood Did Nothing Wrong," Goodwin wrote: "Americans often mistakenly believe organs and tissues are 'free.' Nothing could be further from the truth: Every inch of the human body is financially accounted for . . . These costs include not just charges for harvesting, processing and transportation but also fees for the actual organs."

Aborted babies are only a tiny portion of the billion-dollar biological parts business. "To get an idea of the industry's scale," Goodwin continues, "consider that there are more than 1.5 million human-tissue related surgeries in the United States [and in 2015] 22,000 . . . organ donation surgeries." As noted earlier, the reimbursement to medical institutions, pharmaceutical companies, and physicians is hundreds of thousands to millions for one transplant. Now multiply that by 39,035 for organ transplants in 2020; never mind the other tissue procedures that year or the life-long medical costs—the body parts business is lucrative!

Aborted parts from unwanted babies are just another attempt to increase the donor pool and turn a profit. At least, this is the motive of PP. In fact, increasing the supply of organs in America is favored by ninety-five percent of the population. No woman is forced like those in China or exploited like people in Iran, India, Egypt, or Pakistan. A mother chose to get an abortion, just like a donor made a choice to donate organs. The in-utero baby's remains are harvested for body parts to help others. The mother applies the organ procurement motto to "Give the Gift of Life," just like a registered organ donor under the UDDA.

In December of 2020, *LifeNews.com* published, "Scientists Use Scalps From Aborted Babies to Create 'Humanized Mice' for Research." According to scientists, the research aims to address organ rejection and allow transplants from animals to humans. This is another attempt to increase the donor pool and, yes, to make a profit. The study was funded by the National Institute of Health, our tax dollars.

"The researchers at the University of Pittsburg used 'full-thickness human skin' from babies aborted between 18 and 20 weeks gestation for their experiments, according to their study." *LifeNews.com* continues: "They also took thymus, liver and spleen tissue from aborted babies and 'transplanted and grafted onto rodents and allowed to grow. Then the rodent models were given a staph infection on the skin to study how the internal organs responded,' according to the report."

All of this is grotesque. Nevertheless, it gets to the heart of transplant medicine, which at its core is the removal of a body part from one living creature and transplanting it into another. The biggest challenge is overcoming the rejection, which is why the expense of lifelong anti-rejection drugs is required, even after careful matching with a human donor. Overcoming this barrier will eliminate immunosuppressive drugs and open the door to transplant organs from animals to humans.

In August of 2019, *The Guardian* reported, "Pig to human heart transplant 'possible within three years.'" Pig valves were first used in human heart surgeries in 1968, a process referred to as xenotransplantation. Pigs are the obvious candidates for whole heart surgeries, but something doesn't sit right with the idea of eating a pork chop while a pig's heart beats in one's chest.

Of course, while xenotransplantation, or transplanting animal organs to humans, will lessen the human donor pool's burden, it is filled with obstacles and ethical issues. The primary hurdle is the human rejection of a pig's heart, which is being addressed by harvesting tissue from aborted babies. Aside from cross-transplant ethics, there are also real concerns about raising genetically modified pigs to equip them to be human organ donors.

In 1989, the United States Department of Agriculture (USDA) altered the DNA of pigs by adding genes that produce human growth hormones. The "Beltsville pigs," as they were known, endured visible suffering after the experiment. Even more disturbing is creating a genetically modified human-pig species through rapid cycling to harvest organs. Patricia Piccinini's artwork, *The Young Family*, displayed at the National Museum of Women in the Arts, depicts the tragic halfbreed.

On April 15, 2021, National Public Radio (NPR) aired "Scientists Create Early Embryos That Are Part Human, Part Monkey." According to the article, they were "created in part to try to find new ways to produce organs for people who need transplants." The researchers were motivated by programs like the Beltsville pigs. For this experiment, the scientists decided to use monkeys rather than mice and pigs since their DNA is more closely related to humans. "After one day, the researchers reported, they were able to detect human cells" developing in monkey embryos—abominable.

Organovo, a biological tissue company in California, is trying to create organs with 3D printing to meet organ demand. The technology is still in its infancy, but the researchers believe it will work. A trachea (a windpipe) was recently created for a young girl from her own stem cells. Of course, this structure is significantly less complicated than a kidney, liver, lungs, or a heart.

The "ink" needed to print these 3D organs is from human cells. What better candidates to advance this technology than the immature cells harvested from aborted babies? These infant cells are biologically assigned to specific organs, bones, and tissues. This process may even eliminate problems associated with rejection. A recipient's cells may be mixed into the aborted baby's cells to form the biological "ink" for the 3D printing of a new organ to transplant.

When the demand for organs is high, the supply is low, fear of death is palpable, and the financial rewards are excellent, the greedy and misguided organ procurement business will surge under the cloak of doing the greatest good for society. The narrative from UNOS, OPOs, OTPN, and ninety-five percent of American citizens will be, "we need more organs!" The Christian message is that people need Jesus and his answer for disease and death, not more organs to transplant.

However, considering this organ and tissue harvest hunger and the lucrative prospects, the humanitarian crises worldwide through exploitative red markets, greedy black markets, and oppressive regimes will soar. Attempts to refine xenotransplantation will continue. Murdered unborn babies will be harvested. Hopelessness for those rejecting Jesus and his teaching will persist. These are disturbing matters Christians who "hunger and thirst for righteousness" (Matt. 5:6) need to confront. Still, many Christians ignore everyday evil in the US, and we turn to this homicidal harvest horror next.

3

Legal Death and the Harvest

It was the late 1980s, the decade I (Heidi) missed. That's the standing joke I have with anyone who asks me about television shows like Cheers or awful disasters like the Challenger space shuttle explosion. All physicians know what I'm talking about. After medical school, all aspiring doctors literally "live, move, and have their being" in hospitals. Their lives are consumed with learning how to practice medicine.

After medical school, I started my four-year residency program at a major midwestern university hospital. Like most hospitals connected to universities and large cities, we cared for the sickest of the sick. The medicine practiced at my institution was cutting edge. This was designated a trauma one-level hospital, which meant it was a frequent destination for Life Flights, bewildered and traumatized family members, organ procurement organizations (OPOs), and organ harvests.

Like every other day at work, I arrived at the hospital, changed into my scrubs, and checked in with my supervisor, the attending anesthesiologist. "So far, looks like a quiet night," he said. "There's just an organ harvest that needs to be preop'd. Why don't you go to the ICU and do that?" I suddenly realized this night would not be like any other. I had never been asked to be the anesthesiologist for a brain-dead organ donor.

Quizzically, I looked at my boss. Trying not to sound stupid, I said: "An organ harvest? Is there anything different about this I need to know?"

He looked at me and rolled his eyes. "Just be sure someone has actually declared him brain dead. The transplant team can be a little eager."

Most people assume diagnosing brain death

involves a lot of high-tech equipment. However, tests like an electroencephalogram (EEG), computer tomography (CT) scanning, and magnetic resonance imaging (MRI) are not required by the Uniform Determination of Death Act (UDDA). Sometimes EEGs, CTs, and MRIs confirm bedside findings, but United States (US) law does not mandate their use.

All a person needs are everyday household items, such as a flashlight, cotton swab, turkey baster, and a sewing needle. The diagnosis of brain death under the UDDA requires "accepted medical standards" at the bedside. Which is a routine cardiac, respiratory, and neurological assessment based on clinical judgment.

The donor must not react to outside stimulation. Response to pain may be determined by squeezing a finger or toe, poking the body with a sharp object, or firmly rubbing the patient's breastbone with something hard, like a knuckle. A penlight is used to check how pupils react. The donor's head is turned right and left to test whether the eyes track or remain still, and the eyes are touched with a cotton swab to see if blinking occurs. Ice water is dropped into the ear canal from a syringe to see if the eyes reflexively move.

Then the ventilator is briefly turned off, and the donor is visually monitored for attempts to breathe. This is referred to as the apnea test. Later, we will consider this test in greater detail and the harm it can cause. For now, the mechanics of breathing are in view. After the ventilator is stopped, carbon dioxide in the blood increases, and breathing receptors in the brainstem are expected to respond to cause attempts to breathe. After no visual attempts are made to breathe, the person is declared brain dead. The ventilator is turned back on to stabilize vital signs and to preserve organs.

Dick Teresi, *The Undead*, provides an excellent summary of the neurological criteria for the UDDA. "The logic of brain death goes like this," Teresi writes, "if the brain stem is dead, the higher centers of the brain are also probably dead, and if the whole brain is dead, everything beneath the brain stem is no longer relevant. Since in practice only the brain stem is routinely tested, the vast majority of the body, everything above the brainstem and everything below, no longer counts as human."

Dutifully, I took the elevator up to the intensive care unit (ICU) to perform an assessment on my *"dead"* patient. I found his chart at the nurse's station, sat down, and reviewed it. According to the notes, the twenty-seven-year-old donor was in a motorcycle accident. He sustained a head injury. According to state and federal laws, the ICU physician and neurologist declared him brain dead, so he was legally dead. The OPO received consent from the man's parents to donate his organs.

After closing the chart, I entered the room. I was relieved to find the young man alone. If his family were present, I wasn't sure what I would've said. The canned reassurances, "your son would be kept safe and comfortable during the surgery," didn't seem right. Neither did having the consent form for anesthesia signed. How do you discuss the risks of anesthesia up to and including death with a person who was declared dead? A dead person, no less, still alive with a beating heart! In hindsight, all of it seems so contradictory.

I stepped over to the bedside to examine him.

He looked like most of the trauma patients I had seen. He was warm and pink, monitored, and a ventilator inflated and deflated his lungs. The intravenous (IV) solutions dripped along with air release from the ventilator. The automatic blood pressure cuff inflated and deflated. Illuminated lines on the monitors with beeping sounds traced his heart rhythm, oxygen levels, and arterial pressures. His biological signs of life were stable, at least on the life support.

"He is my age," I said to myself.

After finishing my assessment, I went back to the operating room (OR) area to discuss my plan with the supervising anesthesiologist. I proposed a balanced anesthesia technique involving opioids to control pain and a paralyzing agent to prevent reflex movements during the surgery. My supervisor told me that sounded fine but added, "administer a sedative that causes a loss of consciousness."

Taken back, I looked at him and said, "But

the patient is already dead."

He gazed over his surgical mask, "just in case," and walked away.

The patient was wheeled into the OR connected to life-support. This ensured his organs were not damaged, and several red coolers were brought in. We transferred him to the operating table. I quickly switched him to the ventilator on the anesthesia machine, moved the IV bags to my hangers, and connected the various monitors to my equipment.

I administered the planned anesthesia. The young man's body was shaved, scrubbed with antimicrobial soap, and then draped. As usual, after the surgery started, the patient's heart rate and blood pressure increased. I injected more opioid and a paralyzing agent, and the vital signs returned to normal.

The harvest surgeon cut a vertical line from the neck to the pelvis. Then he used a sternotomy saw, which is like a jigsaw, to cut the sternum or breastbone. The young man's chest cavity was pulled apart with metal retractors to expose his beating heart and lungs, inflating and deflating with the ventilator's help. His heart rate and blood pressure shot up. I gave him more opioid, but his vital signs stayed the same.

Then it dawned on me, "The brain-dead organ donor is responding to slicing, cutting, pulling, and anesthesia!" It was now evident that the man was still alive. Not shortly after this, I injected a high dose of the medication to produce unconsciousness as an act of mercy. *After his beating heart pumped the medicine to his brain, the organ donor's heart rate slowed, and blood pressure lowered.* Then his split-open body was mercilessly ransacked by the harvest surgeon.

While I was busy documenting and trying to make sense of the whole event, the surgeon looked over at me and said, "You can disconnect the ventilator now."

I was startled. "Excuse me?"

"You can turn the ventilator off and go. We're done with you." It was time to deflate the lungs and remove them. I did what the surgeon instructed and turned off the ventilator. As I left, the cooling, perfusing, and organ removal process continued. Outside the OR, I saw more OPO technicians scrubbing up. They were coming to harvest the rest of the body: the young man's corneas, skin, bones, and other tissues.

All of this felt wrong. As a medical doctor who deals with blood and guts, it wasn't the surgery. Others may find the harvest gruesome, but it's a day at the office for a physician. At the time, my conscience was telling me something else was wrong. Most notably, why does a dead person need anesthesia?

Like all medical students, I studied anatomy using a human corpse. My cadaver was cold, stiff, and unresisting. We sliced into her, and nothing happened. However, the organ donor was warm, pink, and responsive. Although the life-support apparatus may account for perfusion, the organ donor's response was something else. Like any other patient I cared for under anesthesia, the young man reacted to the brutal surgical assault on his body.

"Reflexes" is the traditional medical school answer. But a reaction to pain that caused an elevated heart rate and blood pressure was different. This was a stress response occurring between the brain and heart, not a simple reflex. It requires a multi-organ and tissue interaction that includes the nervous and cardiovascular systems. Insensitivity to deep pain is supposed to be one of the defining characteristics of brain death!

Nevertheless, I dutifully followed my medical education and the experts, protected by US law. Even though I saw a person breathing (albeit on a ventilator) with a beating heart. I believed the attending physicians' contradiction of medical science! During the harvest surgery, the donor's biological responses proved what was obvious: *the young man was still alive while being cut apart.* I should've been a medical doctor with a conscience who listened to my gut, followed the science, and was loyal to my oath to do no harm.

Above all, I should have lived up to my commitment as a Christian to seek "first the kingdom of God and his righteousness" (Matt. 6:33), not legal fictions contrary to the law of God (Exo. 20:13). I needed to confess my sin of murder, repent, and ask my heavenly Father for forgiveness.

The UDDA Permits Active Euthanasia

From a scientific standpoint, registered organ donors are not biologically dead. Cellular life, tissues, heart, and integrative (brain and body) life processes continue in these organ donors. The vital organs harvested from these people require continuous perfusion, which means circulation is an absolute necessity. The reality is a registered organ donor never actually crosses the threshold from natural life to death.

The UDDA, which became law in 1981 and permits harvesting organs under the dead donor rule (DDR), defines death thus: "An individual who has sustained either (1) irreversible cessation of circulatory and respiratory functions, or (2) irreversible cessation of all functions of the entire brain, including the brainstem, is dead. A determination of death must be made in accordance with accepted medical standards."

Before its acceptance as law in 1981, the UDDA was controversial. Three presidential councils were appointed to study it: one before its ratification as federal law in 1980, another in 2006, and the other in 2008. The delegations reaffirmed the UDDA while admitting there were inconsistencies. The 2008 committee opted for the term "total-brain failure" instead of "brain death" because it was apparent that brain-dead organ donors had signs of life.

As recently as 2018, Harvard Medical School held "Defining Death: Organ Transplantation and the 50 Year Legacy of the Harvard Report on Brain Death." The conference assembled leading experts in the field, and it was chaired by Dr. Robert Truog. Not one of the leaders saw the UDDA as sufficient to define natural death. The group's consensus: *the UDDA is best viewed as a legal instrument to represent death in the US, not as a way to describe death as a biological occurrence.*

All were agreed that the UDDA raised enormous ethical problems with the DDR. The DDR requires natural death before harvesting organs. "For five decades," writes David Rodriguez-Arias, a contributor, "the DDR has likely contributed to the goal of increasing organ procurement without creating public alarm, but at the same time it has generated a great deal of academic controversy." The experts suggested different ways to address the inconsistencies.

Doctors Franklin Miller and Robert Truog, *Death, Dying, and Organ Transplantation: Reconstructing Medical Ethics at the End of Life*, wrote an entire book about the problem and provided a shocking solution. They write: "As a way of approaching the ideal goal of honest engagement with the legitimacy of vital organ donation from still-living patients, we advocate making these legal fictions transparent by acknowledging that death in the eyes of the law is not the same as death in fact according to a biological definition."

Their answer is to reconstruct medical ethics to permit life termination for organ donors meeting the UDDA criteria. In layman's terms, accept the biological fact that registered organ donors are not dead and perform a Kevorkian style medical mercy killing to ensure they are. According to the doctors, this will respect the organ donor's rights for self-determination, fulfill the DDR requirements, and increase the organ donor pool. It will also eliminate the organ donor's obvious suffering during the harvest surgery, that, I (Heidi) observed first-hand.

At least the doctors are honest, but fundamental questions remain. Consider the young man in the motorcycle accident. Would the parents decide to donate if they knew their son would be deliberately killed to harvest his organs? Better yet, would the organ donor choose to have his organs removed if he knew it would be his demise? We will never know the answer to these questions. However, we know organ donors defined as legally dead in the US still have biological signs of life. Many may even be aware of what's happening during the surgery to remove their organs, and, sadly, some may have even made a full recovery.

Brain Death is NOT Death

Zach Dunlap, a happily married man in his mid-thirties, is raising a family in Oklahoma. In 2007, he suffered a severe head injury after a four-wheeler accident. In a *Dateline* story, his doctor described his injuries as catastrophic. He was pronounced dead according to the UDDA criteria. Zach's license indicated he was a registered organ donor, so the OPO was notified. His organs were scheduled for harvesting.

Zach's cousin, who worked in the medical field, was skeptical of the diagnosis, so he performed a simple bedside neurological exam each time he visited Zach. Then one day, as the cousin ran his closed pocketknife along the base of Zach's foot—his foot moved. Next, he slid an object under his fingernail, and Zach pulled his arm across his body. Finally, he checked to see if Zach's eye responded to light and his pupil constricted. A few days later, Zach was able to tell his family, "I love you," and after forty days in the hospital, Zach was discharged home.

While Zach was "brain dead," a state confirmed by medical technology and professional opinion, he was aware of everything. He said in a 2019 interview with Dr. Paul Byrne: "The next thing I remember was laying in the hospital bed, not being able to move, breathe—couldn't do anything, on a ventilator. I heard someone say, 'I'm sorry he's brain-dead. He's passing away.' And there's nothing I could do, just get mad. I couldn't do anything—to sign—at all. . . . I tried to scream, tried to move, just got extremely angry." Thankfully, the medical professionals listened to Zach's cousin—many don't listen at all.

Jahi McMath, a thirteen-year-old girl from California, made international news after being declared brain dead. In December of 2013, the teen had her tonsils surgically removed at Oakland Children's Hospital. She developed postoperative bleeding and had a cardiac arrest. Jahi was resuscitated and required a ventilator to breathe. According to her doctors, the loss of circulation caused brain death. Three days after her surgery, Jahi was declared legally dead based on the UDDA criteria. She was issued a death certificate.

The family refused to accept she was dead. Byrne advocated for Jahi and her family. After a legal battle, she was released by the hospital and transported to New Jersey. State law in New Jersey allows families to reject a brain death diagnosis if it conflicts with their religious beliefs. Eventually, Jahi was moved to an apartment on a ventilator, had a feeding tube, and received nursing care. As the weeks passed, Jahi started to show signs of responsiveness, which caught the attention of Dr. Alan Shewmon, one of the experts who spoke at the Harvard conference in 2018.

He watched video footage and observed her personally for six hours in her New Jersey apartment. An MRI scan taken nine months after her brain injury showed the brainstem's impairment (the area responsible for regulating the heart and lungs), but it also showed activity in the brain's higher regions. Shewmon determined that Jahi was not dead according to the UDDA; she was in a Minimally Conscious State (MCS), which meant she had a level of awareness.

Then he noted three months after the MRI, "in 2014," now one full year after the tragic event, "the neurologist Calixto Machado studied the heart rate of Jahi McMath and found that it was environmentally responsive—this responsiveness being a clear brainstem function." Now Jahi not only had brain function in her cortex (higher brain), but she also showed signs of recovery in her brainstem (lower brain). Shortly after that, Jahi also started to respond to verbal commands to move.

Shewmon determined these movements were too complex to be reflexes. He noted further that Jahi went through puberty and started menstruating, which requires a functioning hypothalamus (part of the brain). He concluded: at the time of her declaration of death, the bedside neurological examinations, EEGs, and cerebral blood flow studies (CTs and MRIs) could not detect the level of life she possessed. The same was true for Zach.

In October of 2014, an attorney for Jahi's family filed a motion with the California Superior Court requesting a reversal of the legal status of death for Jahi. According to California law, since she was dead, she was not entitled to financial assistance for ongoing care. Shewmon stated in his declaration to the court: "I can assert unequivocally that Jahi currently does not fulfill diagnostic criteria for brain death." Further, "She is an extremely disabled but very much alive teenage girl." Not surprisingly, but sadly, the California court upheld Jahi's death certificate.

According to Shewmon, the instability commonly seen in an acute brain injury will often resolve and stabilize with proper care. In fact, if Jahi was not treated as legally dead at Oakland Children's Hospital, the young teen may have improved even more. The discontinuation of her treatment and lapse of time without hydration, nutrition, and medications may have been harmful to her recovery.

Jahi received her second death certificate five years later in New Jersey. The cause of death on this document was liver failure leading to a cardiac arrest. Jahi was still on the ventilator, had a feeding tube, responded to voices, fellowshipped with her family, and received loving care. According to Dr. James Bernat, another specialist in the field at the Harvard conference, brain death or total brain failure is incorrectly diagnosed sixty-five percent of the time.

Do DCD Donors Really Die?

Before 1981, the only legal way to donate organs in America was five to six minutes after a heart stopped beating. The problem with harvesting organs after heart stoppage is, they may be damaged due to lack of perfusion. It is futile to remove a diseased organ and replace it with a potentially defective one—this defeats the purpose of transplant medicine. This was one of the primary motivators to establish the brain-death standard for death in the first place.

With advances in medical technology, donation after circulatory death (DCD) has re-emerged as another organ source. These people are not brain dead, but they have experienced a severe head or brainstem injury. They're not expected to recover. If these people are registered organ donors or their families consent to donation, they become part of the human body-parts pool.

Under this scenario, the organ donor and family are brought to the OR or a cozy suite nearby. The ventilator and all life support are withdrawn, and the person is monitored until the heart stops beating. Afterward, family members are permitted to wait with the loved one—on average, about two minutes. If the heart does not restart, family members are escorted away, and the bloody harvest begins. At this point, the donor's heart is restarted for the purpose of harvesting organs.

Many physicians are uncomfortable with DCD donation for this reason. I (Chris) worked in an electrophysiology lab at one time. Electrical conduction in the heart is so predictable that, under controlled conditions, it is safe to cause a cardiac arrest and restart the heart. Every day, we shocked (defibrillated) the heart to start it pumping. Often, it took us longer than two minutes to reestablish cardiac function. Nevertheless, these cardiac arrest "victims" were discharged from the hospital later in the day.

What is even more horrific is before defibrillating the heart to restart it in DCD donors, blood flow to the brain is stopped. The reason: *detectable brain function continues*. Studies with EEGs during harvest surgeries documented brain waves. Since brain activity continues in DCD donors, there are legitimate questions of inner awareness or consciousness. But now, due to the plugged blood vessels, the heart cannot pump the anesthesia to the brain to produce unconsciousness! This means the donor experiences the electrical shocks to restart the heart, the harvest cuts, and the pulling apart of his or her chest cavity—barbaric!

A critical care physician, Sam Parnia, conducted two studies on people resuscitated after heart stoppage to evaluate inner awareness. In a five-year multihospital survey of 2,060 cardiac arrest victims, 330 survived, and 142 agreed to be interviewed. Fifty-four people reported consciousness during the resuscitation event. For the remaining eighty-eight questioned, medications and decreased oxygen levels to the brain may have contributed to forgetfulness and memory loss.

In the second study by Parnia in 2019, AWARE II (AWAreness during REuscitation), research captured information beyond awareness. In the hospital where Parnia works, 465 people had cardiac arrests lasting five minutes. Of this group, forty-four survived, and twenty-one agreed to be interviewed. Four reported having personal memories (joy, peace, light, dread, terror, darkness, and encounters with spirit beings), seeing medications administered, and hearing the resuscitation event. AWARE II is still ongoing, but what is obvious is there is more to being human than the brain, heart, and lungs. Thus, DCD donors are not dead!

The UDDA: A Legal Lie

Statements based on law do not always represent reality. For example, the Health Resources & Services Administration says, "Brain death is death and it is irreversible." This is simply not the case, as noted with Zach, Jahi, and most recently Lewis Roberts, a young man in the United Kingdom (UK). Shewmon has documented 175 cases of "brain dead" people who lived after the declaration of death under the UDDA, some for more than twenty years.

According to Truog and Miller, "patients have been legally diagnosed as dead according to the standard criteria, only to begin breathing . . . in the interval between the diagnosis of brain death and the onset of organ procurement." In 2013, *ABC News* reported a brain-dead donor woke up on the operating room table. Recently, the *New York Daily News* reported another similar episode.

I (Chris) had a family acquaintance who suffered from a traumatic brain injury. The young woman tripped, fell, and hit her head on concrete. She was declared dead according to the UDDA, and the OPO representative approached her sister for her organs. She said, "No way!" The ICU physician allowed care for another twenty-four hours. During that time, the woman started to recover. She is walking and talking today.

Lewis Roberts was mentioned above. In March of 2021, Lewis was hit by a van, and he suffered a head injury. He was declared legally dead based on brain-death criteria four days later. Lewis was designated to be harvested, a requirement in the UK, since he did not register as an opt-out organ donor! A few hours before the organ procurement surgery, Lewis became responsive and is recovering today.

An internet search reveals people who were diagnosed dead according to the UDDA and recovered. An Iowa teen, Taylor Hale, suffered a traumatic brain injury in 2011. As her condition worsened, she developed a brain hemorrhage. She was declared brain dead, and her medications and oxygen were removed. Unexpectedly, she started breathing on her own. She was discharged from the hospital and completed high school.

In Texas, George Pickering III suffered a massive stroke. After consulting with George's doctors, his mother and brother decided to withdraw life support, and the local OPO was notified. After George's father found out, he took a stand: "They were saying he was brain dead—he was a vegetable. They were moving too fast." Armed and dangerous, he stood guard over his son. During the standoff in the ICU, George started to respond. "There was a law broken," said George, "but it was broken for all the right reasons. I'm here now because of it."

The UDDA requires "irreversible cessation," but a heart and lungs put into someone else beat and breathe! This is not "irreversible cessation." It is also well-documented that the brain does not cease to function immediately after heart stoppage, as noted above. People whose hearts and lungs have stopped are in the process of dying, but they have not crossed the line from natural life to death. The irreversible switch from biological processes promoting human life in the body to those of death has not been flipped.

Location and a choice impact the irreversible cessation criteria as well. For example, two people may be in identical cardiac arrest situations. Person one, an organ donor, may be harvested in one state in less than five minutes and have his or her organs restarted in someone else. Person two, not an organ donor, can be revived in a different state after five minutes and walk out of the hospital with his or her organs. In both cases, the irreversible cessation standard was not met. The choice and location controlled the outcome, not a universal standard of death.

Aside from this, if a person believes life begins at conception, the heart, lungs, and brain are irrelevant when defining death. Biological death has always been marked by a decrease in cell functions that promote life. Human life started the moment cells came to life in a mother's womb. The reverse must occur for death to be an actual occurrence. There is a biological line between life and death, but it's drawn at the body's cellular level.

In antiquity, natural death was evident to everyone. After a person died, a period of waiting followed to ensure death had occurred. Not only were three days prophesied in the Bible for Jesus, but the elapse of days testified to the public that he was, in fact, dead. Jesus did not experience autoresuscitation or a return of spontaneous circulation (ROSC). He rose from a biologically dead state! Elapsed time without breathing and a heartbeat marked natural death and legal death in the western world until 1968.

However, the shift toward a redefinition of death started in the seventeenth century. As the philosophy of the mind developed, the disciplines of psychiatry and neurology emerged. Eventually, a move away from an immaterial or supernatural spirit giving life to the material or natural body occurred. Specific regions of the brain gained the powers attributed to the person's supernatural part. The brain became the primary and integrative organ necessary for natural life.

In 1747, Julien Offray de la Mettrie published *Man a Machine*. In this influential book, La Mettrie said that human beings "are at bottom only animals and machines." The "soul" or immaterial part, La Mettrie noted, "is but . . . a material and sensible part of the brain, which can be regarded . . . as the mainspring of the whole machine." This is an idea consistent with René Descartes' "ghost in the machine." Supposedly, the brain and the soul or spirit are the same or nearly identical. The body is the brain's mechanical instrument, according to this philosophy.

"In the early 1960s, it was agreed that once the brain stem failed, recovery becomes impossible," wrote Anne Hardy and E. M. Tansey in *The Western Medical Tradition*. They continue: "With this recognition, the development of specific criteria for brain death developed." In 1968, Dr. Henry Beecher published "A Definition of Irreversible Coma" in the *Journal of the American Medical Association*. This article paved the way for the UDDA and a redefinition of legal death, as noted earlier.

In *Death, Dying, and Organ Transplantation*, Miller and Truog comment at length on the biological life signs of people meeting the UDDA criteria and donors under the DDR. Even though they are considered legally dead, the heart continues to beat, blood pressure and heart rate adjust, kidneys produce urine, wounds heal, maturation occurs, hair and nails grow, infections resolve, and healthy babies are delivered.

Yes, a legally dead mother can deliver a living baby, which is not rare. As recently as 2019, a pregnant woman in the Czech Republic had a stroke and was in a brain-dead state for 117 days. On August 15, she delivered a healthy baby girl. The obstetrician said to *Reuters* news, "without [the family's] support and their interest, it would never have finished this way." Sadly, it finished the other way in Texas. The husband of his pregnant brain-dead wife removed life support and killed his unborn baby.

"Drawing on knowledge regarding the functioning of individuals who meet the diagnostic criteria for 'brain death,'" Miller and Truog write, "we contend that they are not dead in accordance with the established biological conception of death in terms of the cessation of the integrative functioning of the organism as a whole." It is *impossible* to establish with scientific certainty, even according to the most advanced and "accepted medical standards," someone has died according to the UDDA.

The gold standard for those on a ventilator is the apnea test. For this examination, a blood sample is taken from an artery (carries oxygen-rich blood to the body). The amount of carbon dioxide in the blood is measured. Then the ventilator is turned off and disconnected. As the carbon dioxide in the arterial blood increases, the person is monitored for breathing (the carbon dioxide in arterial blood stimulates receptors in the brainstem to cause breathing). After the carbon dioxide reaches a certain level in the blood and no visual attempts are made to breathe, a diagnosis of brain death is made.

However, as noted earlier, the reality is that ICU clinicians will often turn off the ventilator and wait. After no spontaneous breathing is observed, they stop the evaluation. They never check to see if the carbon dioxide levels were high enough in the blood to cause the patient to take a breath. Nevertheless, even when the apnea test is appropriately applied, its validity is still questionable. This is due to the harm by the apnea test itself.

Rising levels of carbon dioxide in arterial blood cause dilation or opening of the arteries, contributing to increased blood flow and swelling in the brain. The result is intensified intracranial pressure on the brain enclosed in the skull, which destroys neurons (nerve cells), and this causes stress on the brainstem (where heartbeat and breathing are regulated). The apnea test increases pressure and swelling in the brain, essentially reversing the primary goal for treating a head injury.

Other confounding factors have also contributed to the misdiagnosis of death. Hypothermia must be corrected before death is certified. Many are familiar with amazing stories of survival when people fall through the ice, such as in the 2019 movie, *Breakthrough.* In fact, cooling and warming have become standard features to assist with resuscitation techniques and surgeries.

Most doctors are aware of the need to rewarm the patient before diagnosing brain death. They may not be aware that the brain may need days rather than hours to recover its function after a hypothermic episode. Parnia, the primary investigator in the AWARE studies and author of *Erasing Death,* notes the effects of hypothermia on the body's organs. In his book, Parnia cites reports of people who initially met the criteria for brain death under the UDDA but recovered after being rewarmed.

Parnia writes: "There are in fact case reports of people who had appeared to be brain dead (and had met all the brain death testing criteria) after being examined many hours and days after being warmed up to a normal temperature following hypothermia treatment for cardiac arrest, only to show signs of brain recovery up to seven days later." How many organ donors would've recovered if physicians waited a little longer?

Another insightful statement from the 2018 Harvard conference is from Rodriguez-Arias's presentation, "The Dead Donor Rule as Policy Indoctrination." Referring to a comment by the political science expert Deborah Stone, he says: "policy-making becomes indoctrination whenever public opinions and preferences are intentionally manipulated in ways that destroy or prevent citizens' independent judgment and rational deliberation. . . . The history of death determination in the context of organ donation can be described as an indoctrinating attempt to settle a moral controversy."

That's a rather wordy way of saying, "The public has been deliberately swayed and brainwashed by the UDDA and DDR to address the demands of the harvest elites' craving for transplantable organs!" Shewmon suggests, "Just as cigarette ads are required to contain a footnote warning of health risks, ads promoting organ donation should contain a footnote along these lines: 'Warning: It remains controversial whether you will actually be dead at the time of the removal of your organs.'"

The UDDA and DDR are legal fictions. Harvesting organs from donors defined dead under

US law is a vicious form of active euthanasia. Most importantly, all of this is a great dishonor to the living God, the giver of human life.

4

Life, Death, and the Image of God

I (Chris) think most parents have a baby book for their children. Each one of these books is unique and specific to the child it's about. Usually, the record will have a chronology from conception until birth, reflective entries about the pregnancy, and pictures. In my book about my son, Noah, I have all of these things and more.

I love the picture of him as an infant wrapped in a white blanket with pink and blue stripes. His head is turned to the right, his eyes are closed, and his arms are extended above his head. Every time I look at that picture, it fills my heart with warmth and love. The photo was taken in the hospital a few hours after he was born.

Although not as vivid as this picture, what is

equally precious are the ultrasound pictures I have of him taped in the book. These grainy black and white images with technical information are incredible. "Wow! There's my boy, Noah, not yet fully formed," I say to myself each time I gaze at them. I do more than look; however, I meditate, and my mind is filled with wonder. I recall the days his mother and I sat with the obstetrician at the ultrasound machine.

After squeezing out the cold goop on her protruding belly, the doctor would move the wand around. At some spots, we heard a "whoosh, whoosh" sound. "That's the heartbeat," she said and clicked a button. The obstetrician pointed out Noah's anatomy in the various silhouettes and provided commentary. This was fascinating. What was even more incredible to me was the thought that Noah's life, indeed all human life, started even before I could see him in these images.

In-utero development is a marvel of life, and it is a scientific fact. At the point of conception, a new and separate person is created in a mother's womb, several weeks before consciousness, a heart, brain, or lungs. Life begins at conception. This is not merely a pro-life position; it is a biological reality.

At conception, the new person is a zygote, which is merely a scientific term to explain a stage of development. Other terms used are blastocyst, embryo, fetus, infant, toddler, child, adolescent, adult, and geriatric. What is important to note is a separate person is present throughout each point of growth inside the mother's womb and then outside her in the world. The newly formed zygote in the mother's womb has chromosomes (DNA) from both parents to create a body for human life.

The parent's DNA creates the body, and it has all the properties necessary to begin human development. A biological life process, *apoptosis*, is set into motion after the spirit of God animates the zygote (more on this below). *Apoptosis* will continue until natural death when the spirit of God separates from the body, and another activity called *necrosis* occurs. Via *apoptosis*, which literally means "dropping off," cells are designed to surrender themselves to promote the body's development. This process will continue until systemic *necrosis* or natural death overcomes the body.

After conception, the zygote travels down the fallopian tube, and it divides into a blastocyst. The blastocyst's inner part becomes the embryo (baby), the outer part, the umbilical cord, and the placenta. This is the baby's life support in the womb until, like everyone else, the ongoing necessities of food, water, air to breathe, and dependence on other people are required. *We always need other people and things to survive and are never totally independent for survival.*

At this stage for the helpless baby, embryogenesis starts, cellular differentiation occurs, and the body starts to form. Cells become specific for the cardiovascular tissue (blood, arteries, heart), neurological tissue (nerves, spinal cord, brain), pulmonary tissue (alveoli, bronchial tubes, lungs), etc. These specified cells will perform the physiological processes to sustain the baby's biological life outside the womb.

After three weeks, the baby's heart starts to beat, and blood circulates. In five to six weeks, the spinal cord develops. The brain divides into five different areas, and the cranial nerves emerge. By week eight, the lungs are forming. At this point, all the major bodily structures and physiological systems are present.

Christianity: Life, Death, and Personhood

These are biological truths about natural life. However, medical science is *silent* when explaining how biological tissue comes to life and how we become unique human beings. Theories abound, but all of them are rooted in beliefs — a worldview. Christianity teaches life begins when a unique spirit created by God animates a zygote in a mother's womb to form a distinct person.

Holy Scripture is clear on this teaching (Ps. 100:3; 139:13–16; Isa. 44:24; 64:8; Luke 1:41, 44; 2:6–7). God is the author of life. He creates human life by uniting a supernatural spirit with a natural body composed of elements he already made. Genesis 2:7 is a beautiful portrayal: "the LORD God formed the man from the dust of the ground and breathed into his nostrils the breath of life, and the man became a living being."

The Hebrew word translated as "living being" is *nephesh,* which means "soul." The King James Version translates the "man became a living soul." The Hebrew word for "breath" in "breath of life" is *ruach,* and it also means "spirit." Genesis 1:2: "Now the earth was formless and empty, darkness was over the surface of the deep, and the Spirit (*ruach*) of God was hovering over the waters."

The Old Testament Hebrew scholar William Holladay, *A Concise Hebrew and Aramaic Lexicon of the Old Testament*, says that *ruach* occurs 377 times in the Old Testament. Depending on the context, it means "air in motion, blowing, wind, what is empty or transitory, spirit, mind." In the context of animating a human body, it refers to the *essence* of one's *life* and *personhood*. Also, notice it's one with the soul and body, the "living being."

Human beings are composed of a tight union of created natural elements brought to life at conception by God's supernatural breath to become image-bearers of the Creator of life. The best way to describe biblical thinking on this point is with the term *holistic dualism*. There is a composite of two distinct substances, one natural and the other supernatural. Still, these two are tightly knit together in one unique person, "a living being" or "living soul." At death, Solomon says, "the dust will return to the earth as it was, and the spirit (*ruach*) will return to God who gave it" (Eccl. 12:7).

God's breath of life conferred to a zygote will never cease to exist, nor will the body and soul the spirit animates (more on this below). These are crucial points because the Bible teaches this is true for everyone. There is no annihilationism, unconscious soul sleep, or gnostic dualism (the soul is good, the body is evil)—three pagan beliefs at odds with the Bible. Biological death is not the end!

Death is God's punishment due to Adam's rebellion (Gen. 3:3–4), and we inherited it because we are sinners like him. Paul wrote in Romans: "just as sin entered the world through one man, and death through sin . . . death came to all men, because all sinned . . . the wages of sin is death" (5:12; 6:23). Death is not merely an event at the end of biological life. It is a state of existence and transition point.

Holy Scripture defines death as threefold: spiritual, natural, and eternal. Due to sin, everyone is spiritually dead and appointed to die a biological death. Without spiritual life by faith in Jesus, people will experience eternal death (Rev. 20:6, 14; 21:8). At each appointment with death, the breath of life or spirit will exist. Death here and now is not final, "man is destined to die once," and after natural death, "to face judgment" (Heb. 9:27).

"The man Christ Jesus" (1 Tim. 2:5) sheds crucial light on our human experience in life and death, and as unique individuals created in the image of God. This may seem too obvious to mention, but it's essential to do so. Namely, Jesus the created human was not an afterthought (Eph. 1:3–14). He had a unique and preexistent identity as the second Adam (Rom. 5:12–21).

Even though the divine Son of God always existed, there was a time when the person Jesus did not (Matt. 1:20–21). His human spirit was created and united to a zygote in the *virgin*

Mary's womb (Luke 1:29–33). This is part of the mystery of the incarnation, which is a supernatural event that cannot be fully explained. As a person like us, however, Jesus had a unique identity in his God-breathed spirit.

The same is true for everyone. Our personal identities preexisted in God's mind and were given residence in an essential and precise spirit (cf. Jer. 1:5). God united this unique life-giving spirit to a zygote at conception to bear the Creator's special endowment of human life in time and space. Siegfried Wibbing, in the *New International Dictionary of New Testament Theology,* says, "man's personhood is not something that is at his disposal. It is not founded upon himself. It remains a gift." Is it any wonder the Creator places an infinite price tag on each human being?

Just like Jesus, we share an essential identity that will remain continuous from the womb to the tomb, to a separate state from the body, and back in union with a resurrection body. This is what the Bible teaches about Jesus and, therefore, us (Heb. 4:15). Notice an identity present at conception, without conscious experience, a formed brain, heart, or lungs, and one that will continue without a body after biological death before the body's resurrection.

Unique Human-Spirit Beings

Holy Scripture reveals people who died but re-appeared as spirit beings with their unique identities. Samuel is mentioned in the Old Testament (1 Sam. 28). Moses and Elijah in the Gospels (see Matt. 17:3–8). Others in heaven are mentioned in Hebrews 11 and the martyrs in John's revelation (Rev. 6:9–11). Of course, the Apostles' Creed, "I believe in the communion of the saints," hinges on this teaching of the Bible.

Paul also mentioned being caught up in heaven, "Whether it was in the body or out of the body I do not know—God knows" (2 Cor. 12:2). This experience was more than a vision like John (Rev. 9:17), or Peter's trance (Acts 10:10), or Paul's nightly vision of the Macedonian (Acts 16:9). Paul had an experience where he thought his spirit may have been separate from his body.

There is a sense in which the spirit is locally present with the body, but it also mysteriously transcends it. Aristotelians speak of an ensouled body and Platonists of an embodied soul, but Paul has something different in mind. He talks about a supernatural and natural relationship that cannot be fully explained. Paul's doctrine will be considered later, but the takeaway now is Paul's emphasis on the possibility of having an out-of-body experience (OBE).

According to Plato and Aristotle, natural death follows the soul's separation from the body. Thus, some people define natural death as a lack of conscious experience or a loss of personhood. (The "life unworthy of life" proponents mentioned earlier in the book.) Under these definitions of death, the heart may still beat, but what makes us human has left the body. However, Paul mentions his spirit may be "out of the body" while his body has signs of life. Paul did not see himself as biologically dead or as less than Paul in this separated state.

Doctor Martyn Lloyd-Jones sheds some light on this OBE experience in *Preaching and Preach-*

ers. He mentions the role of "the preacher's own consciousness" during the activity of preaching. During the event, the preacher is outside the body, looking at himself. There is awareness, a consciousness, indeed one's "own consciousness," behind the OBE. This is the testimony of Lloyd-Jones, who reported experiencing this many times. There are also credible reports of OBEs away from the pulpit, especially when people are near death.

I (Chris) recall hearing a story of a woman who had a cardiac arrest. During the resuscitation event, one of the nurses ran into a different room to get medication. She needed to break the glass ampule's top with her thumb to draw out the drug with a syringe. The nurse cut her thumb in the process. After the woman was revived, she suggested the nurse use a face cloth the next time she breaks an ampule. When questioned, the woman said she saw her cut her thumb in a room with medications in it.

Parnia, who was mentioned earlier, has studied near-death experiences (NDEs) for many years. In five years of research, which is still ongoing, he has found consistent themes among cardiac arrest victims who were resuscitated. Parnia questioned these people about their experiences without a beating heart. The individuals reported memories of the resuscitation and other occurrences mentioned in the last chapter.

Parnia mentioned a man who had a cardiac arrest in the hospital's catheterization lab. This is where the vessels (coronary arteries) around the heart are treated. He experienced ventricular fibrillation (the heart stops beating and quivers) during the procedure and went unconscious. According to his medical records, he required two shocks to restart his heart. After he was revived, Parnia questioned him. The man recalled hearing someone say: "Shock the patient, shock the patient." He also reported that he was looking down at the doctor and nurse resuscitating him.

In 2011, doctors in Canada reported a young pregnant woman who became short of breath while giving birth. She was diagnosed with an ascending aortic dissection. The aorta is the major blood vessel coming out of the heart that provides oxygen-rich blood to the brain and body. A dissection is a rupture or split in a blood vessel. Depending on the dissection's size and location, a quick death from internal bleeding may follow. The mother's condition was critical.

After the baby was delivered via c-section, the mother had surgery to repair the ascending aorta. Since her operation was emergent, she did not see or talk to the surgical team. She was administered general anesthesia after the delivery, and her eyes were taped shut before entering the operating room (OR). According to *resuscitation-journal.com*, she saw the OR, herself on the table, the surgical nurse, and the cardiothoracic surgeon. She also described the anesthesia and perfusion machines.

Teresi, who we met earlier, mentioned the account of a woman, Pam, who underwent a brain procedure using hypothermic cardiac arrest. During this type of surgery, the body temperature is lowered to sixty degrees Fahrenheit by running it through a heart-lung cooling machine. After the body is sufficiently cooled, the heart and lungs are stopped. The cooling preserves the body, and the lack of blood flow permits brain surgery.

During the procedure, Teresi reported that the electroencephalogram (EEG) showed no electrical activity in the brain for five minutes, but Pam still had awareness. She remembered hearing the high-pitched whine of the bone saw cutting her skull, and she reported being outside her body. "I looked (down) at my body and knew it was mine, but I didn't relate to it being me."

Pam described the surgical instruments, the heart-lung machine, and even the music played in the OR. She accurately reported the conversations taking place amongst the surgical staff. Pam's OBE is fascinating because she was fully monitored and documented to have no beating heart, respiratory function, or brain activity. Interestingly, first century Christians and Jews believed the spirit was still present with the body for a period after breathing stopped, and it could even reanimate it.

If anything at all, NDEs and OBEs should cause us to pause and exercise caution when determining biological death. While there is a close association between the body-soul and spirit, the breath of God permits unique perceptions consistent with one's identity distinct from the "living being." After all, God's breath of life is supernatural and not subject to natural laws! This is a mysterious relationship. As Paul says, "God knows," and we don't.

Two States, One Person, and Jesus' Victory

While Paul willingly admits ignorance before God and has material in his teaching "hard to understand" (2 Peter 3:16), he has a great deal to say about the human body. The Greek word for body is *soma*, and it's profitable to stick with the Greek when Paul uses it. Paul does not have in mind a body as distinct from a soul, like Plato or Aristotle. Instead, Genesis 2:7 forms his thinking. Paul means a body-soul union as a "living being" or "living soul" when he uses *soma*.

Wibbing mentions three significant themes in Paul's thinking about *soma*. First, there is a somatic or bodily existence. The *soma* (even at conception) testifies to the holistic person's presence, a union of soul-body and breath of life. Second, the *soma* is the essential person. One's identity in the spirit is one with the body and soul. Third, the present *soma* and the resurrected *soma* are the same individual. The difference is the state of existence, not a transformation of substance.

A person's God-breathed spirit in Paul's understanding, Wibbing says, "is thinkable only in a body . . . an earthly or 'physical body' and a 'spiritual body.'" Either a *soma psychikon* or *soma pneumatikon*. Paul uses these same terms in 1 Corinthians 15 when he talks about the end-time resurrection of the body.

He writes: "it is sown a natural body, it is raised a spiritual body. If there is a natural body, there is also a spiritual body. So it is written: 'The first man Adam became a living being'; the last Adam, a life-giving spirit. The spiritual did not come first, but the natural, and after that the spiritual" (vv. 44–50). The emphasis is not on substance (natural and spiritual), but on states of existence, as a natural body (*soma psychikon*) and spiritual body (*soma pneumatikon*).

The Greek suffix *ikon* is the root word *ikos*, an adjective describing the *psyche* (soul or mind) and *pneuma* (spirit) as a state of existence—an "icon" or image-bearer of the Creator of life in two states of being as a person. Paul says it is like being "unclothed" at one time and "clothed" at another (2 Cor. 5), but it's the same person who was naked (a natural body) and dressed (a spiritual body). The *soma psychikon* represents a present body as an image-bearer of the living God. The *soma pneumatikon* is a Christian's future body in the likeness of Jesus' resurrected body— a glorified image-bearer of the living God.

Today, many Christians embrace concepts about the body, spirit, soul, and mind rooted in pagan philosophy. These beliefs influence the way Christians make choices about donating organs. For example, I (Chris) have been at the bedside of numerous non-responsive people with beating hearts. I've heard Christians say things like, "Our son left us after the accident," and make a medical decision based on that belief. This is not God's teaching through the apostle Paul. It's a view of the body and spirit or soul tied to Plato or Aristotle.

Paul teaches that if biological signs of life are present in the *soma*, a holistic body and soul union exists. The child is still a living person. His unique identity in the God-breathed spirit is present with his body. The same is true for elderly parents with dementia or others with severe mental incapacity. These people still bear the image of God (more on this below). Wibbing notes, "It is un-Pauline to think of the body merely as a figure or form," which is Greek philosophy. Citing Romans 6:12 and 12:1, Wibbing says: "the *soma* is not merely an outer form but the whole person." Paul does not have in mind "any division of man into soul and body along the lines of pagan anthropology."

Recall how some of the philosophers at Athens dismissed Paul when he mentioned the resurrected *soma* of Jesus (Acts 17:22–32). The elites referred to Paul as a bird picking seeds out of manure! Those who mocked him believed the ideal state was a *psyche* or soul separated from the *soma*, but Paul taught the opposite. Paul's Greek *psyche* is parallel with the Hebrew *nephesh* (soul). Which refers to the person's present state as "a living being" or a body-soul in union with a God-breathed spirit (Gen. 2:7).

God created Adam's body from the earth, breathed life into it, and Adam became a *soma psychikon*. While living in this natural body, Adam rebelled against God's command. As a result, he died spiritually and was appointed to die biologically. The second Adam (see 1 Cor. 15; Rom. 5) came into the world as a *soma psychikon*. He did so to obey the triune Creator and suffer the penalty for sin—death in its threefold manifestation: spiritual, biological, and eternal (2 Tim. 1:7–10). Jesus conquered sin and rose from the grave victorious over death as a *soma pneumatikon*.

The continuity between both bodies lies in God's breath of life, not the present *psyche* or the future *pneuma*. Paul's teaching is "influenced by Jewish anthropology," notes Wibbing, which is *holistic dualism*. "The body, in the sense of the 'I,' the 'person,' will survive death through the creative act of God." The "creative act" refers to the life-giving spirit from the Creator in union with a zygote (*soma*) at conception, making each person a unique image-bearer of God until biological death.

Natural death causes a temporary division between the *soma* and God-breathed spirit. While this doctrine is taught throughout Holy Scripture, Jesus' death serves as the best illustration. He breathed his last and gave up the spirit (Matt. 27:50; John 19:30). After he died, his body lay lifeless for three days in the tomb, but his spirit continued to live. He said to the repentant criminal on the cross, "today you will be with me in paradise" (Luke 23:43-46). Jesus had a *soma* and spirit separation after natural death because of sin (2 Cor. 5:21).

According to Holy Scripture, Jesus lay in the grave for three days. This period is essential. Not only was it the lapse of time prophesied by Jesus (Matt. 12:40), but it also certified death had taken place. Jesus was biologically dead, and he rose from this state of natural death victorious over the "wages of sin" (Rom. 6:23). His death was a historical and biological fact, and his resurrection a reality.

After a lethal illness, disease, or trauma overcomes the body's biological processes to cause heart and lung failure, natural death or systemic *necrosis* occurs shortly after that. What follows is decomposition due to the lack of circulation and oxygen. What happens next is putrefaction, purging, and decay over time, where the tissues of the body liquefy and return to the earth to become elements for recycling—the "dust" of Holy Scripture.

According to God's will, transplant medicine is a moral, ethical, and honorable pursuit for this reason. Of course, provided people are not murdered, prostituted, or exploited! God created the material world *ex nihilo* to be a closed system. "God saw all that he had made, and it was very good" (Gen. 1:31). In the renewed creation, the old, "very good," material creation will continue. Presumably, natural laws like *apoptosis* will persist, but there will be no sin, disorder, death, or *necrosis*. According to Holy Scripture, the resurrected body will consist of these mysteriously reassembled subatomic particles that are constantly recycled.

The natural body and what we do with it is just as important to the Creator as the supernatural spirit. Those who reject Jesus will not have a *soma pneumatikon*. Since these people despised God's image in life, they will no longer bear it after biological death. Nevertheless, they will still rise from the dead in some type of resurrected body. "For we must all appear before the judgment seat of Christ," says Paul, "that each one may receive what is due him for the things done while in the body, whether good or bad" (2 Cor. 5:10).

Apparently, these "objects of wrath" will now fully bear the image of Satan (Rom. 9:22), to whom these unfortunate people gave their spiritual allegiance to in life (Eph. 2:2). Now they are forever lost to healing, eternal life, and to a body without suffering. These sad souls will exist in a state of eternal death, and they will experience an awful type of everlasting dying, without any mercy and hope (Luke 16:19–31). Take heed, "for your lifeblood I will surely demand and accounting," says the Creator of life, as well as "an accounting for the life of another human being"

(Gen. 9:5).

Returning to the ancient practice of waiting three days to declare natural death would protect human life and honor the Creator who gives it. The deceased's body was "watched" or laid in a tomb in antiquity to ensure death had arrived. The remnants of watching, historically the *vigilia*, are somewhat preserved in the modern-day wake. In historic Christianity, the vigil started two to three days before a deceased believer was commemorated and committed to the ground—the funeral.

Sometimes we hear about people waking up in morgues or in body bags. In 2017, *Medical News Today* published an article written by Honor Whiteman about the Lazarus syndrome. These people experienced auto resuscitation. Most of those written about did so after ten minutes of heart stoppage. About half of the group recovered without significant impairment. Recall, most donation after circulatory death (DCD) donors in the US are harvested after a mere two minutes!

The article opened with a ninety-one-year-old woman who woke up in a hospital morgue eleven hours later "with a craving for tea and pancakes." It goes on to cite numerous cases of the phenomenon occurring in others. In October of 2020, *LifeNews.com* reported the discovery of a living twenty-three-week-old baby in a morgue fridge. In antiquity, the three-day "watch period" and care of the body ensured death was a scientific fact. It was also a part of the grieving process for closure.

Christians should not be hasty to enclose in small spaces, embalm, incinerate, or bury people declared dead. A waiting period is necessary to ensure natural death has occurred, confirm God's breath of life will no longer animate the *soma*, and to help with the heartache associated with loss. The only factual definition of biological death is elapsed time without cardiopulmonary function. This is the biblical standard, nothing less.

The UDDA Devalues the Image of God

Perhaps, one of the greatest tragedies in Christendom today is the acceptance of the Uniform

Determination of Death Act (UDDA) as a definition of death. As noted, numerous times throughout the book, the reality is people meeting the UDDA criteria are not biologically dead. Christians affirming this legal fiction do not see God's image in the animating spirit a zygote receives at conception, no matter what they profess to believe. They see God's image in attributes, such as the ability to reason, exercise virtue, or possess consciousness, but not in Paul's *soma psychikon* doctrine.

Consider Tom, a person in a persistent vegetative state (PVS) since birth, who I (Chris) cared for several years ago. He was put on a ventilator after he was born. Shortly after, a difficult decision was made to withdraw it. Tom was supposed to experience biological death, but he breathed on his own. Since that day, he lay nonresponsive in his bed with a beating heart. There was not a day in Tom's life he exhibited any of the attributes mentioned above.

Tom was about four feet from head to toe when I met him in his late teens, and his physique was mangled. He had a twisted spine, hunched back, an enormous head, and a dispro-portioned body. He had no coordinated move-ments in his limbs; in fact, both of his arms were flaccid and limp. Tom's hands were contracted, and his legs were stiff. His left leg was longer than his right, and his foot was turned back onto his shin.

Some would judge Tom's life as a life not worth living. Tom was not easy to look at. People would turn their gaze away from him in shock, awkwardness, and disgust. Many saw Tom as possessing no "potential" and as a finan-cial burden to taxpayers. For those dedicated to the Beecher doctrine, Tom had a "life unworthy of life," and he deserved to be put out of his *presumed* misery and harvested for organs and tis-sues!

Aside from his apparent deficiencies and need for nursing care, Tom's body still func-tioned to sustain life. What was patently obvious to me, even in this non-responsive state with complete dependence on others, Tom was *alive*, and he was a *person*. More importantly, he had a specific type of life. *Tom was a unique individual with the life-giving spirit of God, minus the ability to reason, exercise virtue, or exhibit conscious behavior.* Tom lived for twenty years in this *soma psychikon* state.

People like Tom are on a slippery slope, and, of course, at present, unresponsive donors with beating hearts have slipped to the bottom. The Bible is clear about life beginning at conception, and all faithful Christians defend this pro-life conviction. Holding this position affirms that life starts several weeks before the brain, heart, lungs, and consciousness develop. This raises the question: "Did the Bible ever teach the image of God was in anything other than the breath of life a zygote receives from the Creator?" The answer, if a Christian wants to be consistent, must be "no."

The image of God is human life itself and not anything else. "He is the living God," wrote Jeremiah (10:10). It is the character of the supernatural and natural livingness God breathes into everyone that makes humans bear God's image, no matter what condition the body is in. It is human life itself, or, instead, him- or herself (cf.

John 1:1–4). "Then God said, 'Let us make man in our image, in our likeness' " (Gen. 1:26). There is an essential distinction between "image" and "likeness" in this passage.

The difference is between God-breathed perfection or God-breathed life to define God's *soma psychikon* in everyone. Each person bears the Creator's image. He or she has a *unique identity* and *life*, a God-breathed spirit. After the Fall, only Jesus possessed the God-breathed likeness of the Creator. However, now Jesus' Holy Spirit inspired *soma psychikon* disciples can strive after the divine likeness by honoring all image-bearers of God! "Be perfect," said Jesus regarding the mercy of the triune Creator for *everyone* at this present day and age, "as your heavenly Father is perfect" (Matt. 5:48).

The sixth commandment is clear: "You shall not murder" (Exo. 20:13). A Christian's baptism, a profession of faith, church attendance, doctrinal knowledge, or excitement in worship are of little value in the Creator's eyes when the breath of life he gives is not cherished. Divine image-bearers who live in the Creator's likeness value human life, no matter how substantially diminished that life may be. Christians endorsing the UDDA don't. Aborting a zygote at conception is murder in God's eyes. So is removing organs from legally dead donors with signs of biological life.

Conclusion:
Life in the Spirit with the Spirit of Life

Much of the Christian life here and now is living with a proper perspective. When it comes to *Harvesting Organs & Cherishing Life*, fundamental to this view and way of living is Jesus' approach to disease, healing, and death. Jesus, not medical science, has "abolished death," and he has "brought life and immortality to light through the Gospel" (2 Tim. 1:10, KJV). This Christian viewpoint has not changed in the twenty-first century (Heb. 13:8).

Nevertheless, commitment and trust in the abilities of modern medicine have undervalued Jesus' triumph as the Resurrection and the Life for many Christians in our era. Today, this is seen in an aggressive pursuit for healing to avoid death at all costs. Christians in the first century had this struggle too. After all, who wants to get sick and die or see a loved one suffer and go to the grave? No one, not even the most stalwart Christian, but this real human struggle does not permit making Jesus' answers to disease, healing, and death secondary to medical science.

A profoundly human and real-life experience is Jesus raising Lazarus from a biologically dead state as a *sign* for everyone to embrace. This first-century encounter encapsulates the message of our book and the perennial struggles people encounter when faced with disease and death. The story also anticipates how people will respond to what we wrote in *Harvesting Organs & Cherishing Life*.

Before digging into the account in John 11, a brief comment about a *sign* and its relationship to a miracle. Jesus' healing and resurrection miracles were pointers aimed at him as the *only* hope in life and death. These *signs* testified to Jesus' supernatural control over the natural order and the I AM claims recorded throughout John's Gospel. I AM the Resurrection. I AM the Life. This is the message of John 11.

Jesus and the Creator of life are one. John says the *signs* Jesus performed were "written that you may believe that Jesus is the Christ, the Son of God, and that by believing you may have life in his name" (20:31). This teaching is fundamental to Christianity. The *sign* of Lazarus's resurrection recorded in John 11 points us back to the famous new birth or first resurrection discourse in John 3.

The resurrection Jesus was speaking about in this passage was not merely a future occurrence; it was a present reality. As John said in Revelation 20:6: "Blessed and holy are those who have part in the first resurrection. The second death has no power over them." This is a resurrection from spiritual and eternal death, along with the promise of a future bodily resurrection from a biologically decomposed state.

It is faith in Jesus as the Resurrection and the Life that looks forward in hope for physical healing at his second coming. At present, those who believe in Jesus "shall not perish but have eternal life" (John 3:16). This is the first resurrection, and it is also a prerequisite to becoming a *soma pneumatikon* at the second.

The Lazarus event recorded in John 11 can be broken up into three sections: Jesus allows Lazarus to die (vv. 1—16), Jesus comforts Lazarus's sisters (vv. 17—37), and Jesus reverses Lazarus's biologically dead state (vv. 38—44). Embedded within this encounter are the real-life battles Christians face and how various groups reacted to Jesus.

The account opens with Jesus and the disciples receiving the sad news that "Lazarus was sick" (v. 1). "Lord, the one you love is sick" (v. 3). Sorrowful news indeed, and the world is filled with it because of the Fall. One cannot listen to the news without hearing about those sick and dying with COVID-19. Christians will always receive reports about disease and death until the first resurrection comes to fruition in the second.

After the news about Lazarus's illness, John provides background information. Lazarus is Mary and Martha's brother, and he lives in Bethany, which is only two miles from Jerusalem. Recently Jesus had threats made to his life in this region. Then John zooms in on Mary. "This Mary," John writes, "whose brother Lazarus now lay sick, was the same one who poured perfume on the Lord and wiped his feet with her hair" (v. 2).

John's point is Mary adores Jesus, and this sets the scene for her later appearance in John 11. At this penultimate summit, Jesus is deeply moved in different ways, and then the powerful climax of Lazarus's resurrection follows. Mary serves as an essential catalyst for Jesus' divine and human response and as a bridge to the resurrection event. At that point in the encounter with Mary, John displays the dual natures of Jesus as the Creator of life and as a person with God's breath of life.

Jesus Allows Lazarus to Die

Lazarus must have died shortly after the messengers left Bethany, which accounts for the four days he was in the tomb (v. 39). One day for the journey of the messengers to reach Jesus. Then Jesus remained where he was for two days, and the one day it took him to travel to Bethany. It would be sure to everyone that Lazarus was dead. Therefore, this *sign* will confirm Jesus' power to grant spiritual and eternal life here and now and the Christian's final victory over disease and death at his second coming.

After Jesus heard the report from the sisters, he replied to the messengers in the presence of the Twelve. "This sickness will not end in death. No, it is for God's glory so that God's Son may be glorified through it" (v. 4). The Twelve probably thought about the blind man Jesus recently healed with mud, spit, and water from the Pool of Siloam.

John writes about that event: "Rabbi, who sinned, this man or his parents, that he was born blind? 'Neither this man nor his parents sinned,' said Jesus, 'but this happened so that the work of God might be displayed in his life'" (9:2–3). While disease and death are awful tragedies associated with the Fall, they are ultimately linked to God's eternal purposes. For Christians back then and for those today, their diseases "do not end in death." All of them, in a *mysterious* way, are ultimately "for God's glory so that God's Son may be glorified" (11:4).

Jesus is not glorified when his perspective on disease and death is not central in the Christian's life. Not because he's arrogant, but because every other view is ultimately aimed at Satan, no matter how compassionate, hopeful, and honorable it appears. "And no wonder," writes Paul, "for Satan himself masquerades as an angel of light" (2 Cor. 11:14). In the end, medical science and healing miracles fail, and people die. Neither can modern medical guidance be relied on, especially considering its perspective on modern organ harvesting practices.

At the heart of making modern medical decisions for Christians is Jesus' viewpoint. Christians need to ask themselves: "Is Jesus and his teaching at the center of my choice to donate or receive an organ? Is the work Jesus accomplished on my behalf directing my life?" If Jesus' perspective isn't, Satan's is. There is no middle ground.

Based on Jesus' statement in John's account about Lazarus, the Twelve probably thought Jesus knew Lazarus would get well, and they were relieved (John 11:12). After all, Jesus sent the messengers away and stayed behind (v. 6). Two days later, they were surprised to hear Jesus say, "Let us go back to Judea" (v. 7). The Twelve were not fond of the idea, "But Rabbi," they said, "a short while ago the Jews tried to stone you, and yet you are going back there?" (v. 8).

Jesus answered them with a cryptic statement. He says, "Are there not twelve hours of daylight? A man who walks by day will not stumble, for he sees by this world's light. It is when he walks by night that he stumbles, for he has no light" (v. 9). In antiquity, there were twelve hours to a workday. People worked from morning to evening, and Jesus had work to do in Judea, regardless of the risks.

Jesus was not afraid to die, and neither should a Christian fear death if it's according to God's will. When Christians live in the power of Jesus' resurrection, they will trust him. If a professing believer has an excessive fear of death, Jesus says the person needs to examine if he or she is a Christian. "A man who walks by day will not stumble," Jesus says, "for he sees by this world's light. It is when he walks by night that he stumbles, for he has no light"—no light for Jesus means no spiritual life (see 1 John 1:6).

"After he had said this, he went on to tell them, 'Our friend Lazarus has fallen asleep; but I am going there to wake him up.' His disciples replied, 'Lord, if he sleeps, he will get better.' Jesus had been speaking of his death, but his disciples thought he meant natural sleep.' So then he told them plainly, 'Lazarus is dead, and for your sake I am glad I was not there, so that you may believe. But let us go to him'" (John 11:11–15).

The work Jesus had to do was to go to the hostile region of Judea to "wake" Lazarus up. Back then, the phrase "fallen asleep" was a common euphemism for death. Nevertheless, the disciples thought Lazarus was sick, and rest would heal him. However, the Twelve should've put two and two together: "fallen asleep" as dead and "wake him up" as resurrection. Jesus clarifies: "Lazarus is dead, and for your sake I am glad I was not there, so that you may believe. But let us go to him."

When it comes to Jesus' ability to raise the dead, the Twelve were not in total darkness. Before the resurrection of Lazarus, the apostles were eyewitnesses to Jesus' raising of Jairus's daughter from a biologically dead state (Luke 8:40–56), as well as the son of the widow at Nain (7:11–15). Nevertheless, the Twelve did not recall these two resurrection *signs*, and they thought rest would heal Lazarus. After all, Jesus did not rush off to see him.

It seems insensitive that Jesus would be glad to be absent from Lazarus while dying. Besides knowing what he would do at Lazarus's tomb as a *sign*, it was not cold from Jesus' perspective. He believed in the present reality of the first resurrection, new birth to eternal life, and the ongoing spiritual communion of believers after biological death. A Christian's disease never ends in death but only in sleep, and the God-breathed spirit continues to live.

These were not mere confessional statements Jesus made; they were living doctrines that permeated his spirit, formed his worldview, and motivated his behavior. This was Jesus' perspective about life and death. Christians may look at many proofs to see how they walk with Jesus, like whether they fear death or hold to correct doctrine. Still, there is only one genuine mark for a true Christian: *commitment to Jesus and his perspective, regardless of doubts, questions, and confusion. This is the one absolute character trait of every Christian back then and today.*

Notice what the Twelve do. Regardless of their lack of understanding, insecurity, and fear of death, they follow Jesus to Bethany. Even with the real possibility of being stoned, the disciples go with Jesus anyway. The Twelve willingly follow him, regardless of the consequences. Is this how you walk with Jesus? Are you committed to him and his teaching at all costs? Along the way, they are met by Lazarus's sister.

Jesus Comforts Lazarus's Sisters

Martha says some remarkable things to Jesus, but her grief causes a lack of trust in the present power of Jesus as the Resurrection and the Life. Martha says to him, "I know that even now God will give you whatever you ask" (11:22). Martha, however, didn't think a present bodily resurrection for Lazarus was in the asking! Like the Twelve, Martha is confused about the first resurrection, new birth to eternal life, as well as Jesus' supernatural ability to reverse biological death.

"For just as the Father raises the dead and gives life," Jesus said earlier in John's Gospel, "even so the Son gives life to whom he is pleased to give it" (5:21). This claim is significant, as we will see in Jesus' later encounter with Martha. Aside from the materialistic Sadducees, who denied the possibility of lifeless people rising from the dead, the rest of the Jews believed God alone possessed the power of resurrection. In John 5, Jesus claimed to have a supernatural power God alone had.

Jesus said to Martha, "'Your brother will rise again.' Martha answered, 'I know he will rise again in the resurrection at the last day.' Jesus said to her, 'I am the resurrection and the life. He who believes in me will live, even though he dies; and whoever lives and believes in me will never die. Do you believe this?' 'Yes, Lord,' she told him, 'I believe that you are the Christ, the

Son of God, who was to come into the world'"
(11:23–27).

Martha's affirmation of an end-time resurrection of the dead is in keeping with Jesus' own teaching (6:39–44, 54) and that of the Pharisees (Acts 23:8). Martha knows her doctrine, but grief has hindered her present trust. Notice what Jesus says and Martha doesn't. Jesus said to her, "I am the resurrection and the life. He who believes in me will live, even though he dies; and whoever lives and believes in me will never die. Do you believe this?" (John 11:25–26). Martha answered yes but notice not with a *confident* yes to Jesus as the Resurrection and the Life.

The emphatic "I am" in "I am the resurrection and the life" points back to Exodus 3:14 and Moses's encounter with God. In this *numinous* passage, the glorious triune Creator says to Moses from a bush burning with holy fire: "I AM WHO I AM." In other words: The infinite, eternal, self-existent, and all-powerful Creator of life is speaking to you! Jesus is essentially saying to Martha, "I am not merely a divine healer. I AM WHO I AM is standing before you!" Jesus and the Creator of life are one. "He who believes in me will live," like Lazarus, "even though he dies; and whoever lives and believes in me will never die," like Lazarus again!

The Twelve are confused, afraid, and uncertain, and Martha is grieving like someone who has no hope. The first-century Christians struggle with trust in the reality of the first resurrection and how this present truth relates to eternal life here and now. The disciples do not understand how Jesus' victory over sin relates to their current triumph over disease and death. Satan, the great deceiver, is at work to inspire chaos and hopelessness. With all of this going on, Mary, full of despair, arrives.

Mary says essentially the same thing as mournful Martha, "Lord, if you had been here, my brother would not have died" (John 11:32, 21). It's as if the two heartbroken sisters repeated a similar saying over and over while Lazarus was in the throes of dying, hoping Jesus would've arrived to heal him. Perhaps, the sisters are even criticizing him for not coming sooner to cure the one he supposedly loved (v.

3). The two sisters focus on Jesus as a divine healer to provide ongoing life here and now, not as the Resurrection and the Life for spiritual and eternal life.

At this point, divine wrath merges with holy anger in Jesus' bosom toward sin, Satan, death, and lack of trust. Jesus was "deeply moved in spirit and troubled" (v. 33). The Greek phrase literally means he was possessed with raging anger, and he was ready to attack. The image is a ferocious and courageous soldier about to clash in battle. Jesus was full of righteous rage toward the causes of human suffering and, yes, the disciple's lack of implicit trust in him as the answer for disease and death. He hates sin in all its forms. Distrusting Jesus is to trust Satan!

In Matthew's Gospel, shortly after Peter confessed Jesus was the "Christ, the Son of the living God" (16:16), Peter was sternly rebuked. After he praised Peter's confession, Jesus talked about how he must suffer, die, and rise from the dead on the third day. Peter challenged Jesus' implicit trust in his Father's will for him, and this incensed Jesus.

Matthew wrote: "Jesus turned and said to Peter, 'Get behind me, Satan! You are a stumbling block to me; you do not have in mind the things of God, but the things of men'" (v. 23). Jesus then went on to talk about the cost of being a Christian: "If anyone would come after me, he must deny himself and take up his cross and follow me. For whoever wants to save his life will lose it, but whoever loses his life for me will find it" (vv. 24–25).

According to Jesus, *commitment* to him and his teaching is a necessary first step for a Christian, but he also requires absolute *trust*. Divided allegiances infuriate Jesus because they hinder the Christian's ability to live according to the Father's will for him or her. They open the door to demonic influences, confusion, despair, fear of death, and grasping after ungodly solutions like unethical modern organ harvest practices!

Yet, Jesus is still full of empathy toward those committed to him and his teaching. "'Where have you laid him?' he asked. 'Come and see, Lord,' they replied. Jesus wept" (John 11:33–35). A better translation for "Jesus wept" is he burst into tears. John puts the full humanity of Jesus on display in a profoundly emotional way in this encounter with Mary. As Isaiah prophesied long ago, "Surely he took up our infirmities and carried our sorrows" (53:4; see also Matt. 8:17; Heb. 2:18; 4:15).

Jesus Raises Lazarus from the Dead

"Jesus, once more deeply moved, came to the tomb. It was a cave with a stone laid across the entrance. 'Take away the stone,' he said" (John 11:39). Weeping Jesus still raging with anger attacks, but not before Martha reminds him Lazarus's dead body was starting to decompose. I suspect Jesus looked at sorrowful Martha with a tender eye and Satan with a piercing gaze of fury. In a voice of divine wrath, righteous anger, and empathy, he said to Martha: "Did I not tell you that if you believed, you would see the glory of God?" (John 11:40).

Jesus told Martha that he was the Resurrection and the Life. She even confessed: "I believe that you are the Christ, the Son of God, who was to come into the world" (v. 27). Nevertheless,

Martha still does not trust Jesus' supernatural power over death as the Creator of life. She was not alone—no one at the tomb had implicit trust in Jesus as the Resurrection and the Life.

Notice what Jesus does and says after the tomb is opened. As the stench of Lazarus's rotting corpse wafts from the black hole, "Jesus looked up and said, 'Father, I thank you that you have heard me. I knew that you always hear me, but I said this for the benefit of the people standing here, that they may believe that you sent me" (vv. 41–42). Recall Martha's earlier words to Jesus: "I know that even now God will give you whatever you ask" (v. 22).

Even though the Son and the Father are one supernatural being (10:30), the person, Jesus, sent by the Father, looked up and prayed. Then "in a loud voice," Jesus shouts, "'Lazarus, come out!' The dead man came out, his hands and feet wrapped with strips of linen, and a cloth around his face. Jesus said to them, 'Take off the grave clothes and let him go'" (11:43–44). "For just as the Father raises the dead and gives life, even so the Son gives life to whom he is pleased to give it" (5:21). Jesus was pleased to give it to Lazarus as a *sign* so others would believe he is the Resurrection and the Life back then and today.

How Various Groups Reacted to Jesus

The first-century reactions recorded in John 11 are perennial. These are also modern responses we anticipate toward *Harvesting Organs & Cherishing Life*. Some people will be angry, dismissive, and offended by what we wrote, and others will consider *Harvesting Organs* with a sincere and reflective heart.

After the famous "Jesus wept" passage in John 11:35, there were two emotionally driven responses: "the Jews said, 'See how he loved him!' But some of them said, 'Could not he who opened the eyes of the blind man have kept this man from dying?'" (vv. 36-37). The people in these two groups are motivated by feelings and emotions. The first by sentimentalism and the second by pessimism; both groups passed a judgment on Jesus.

Driven by their opinions about Jesus, they never come to know Jesus for who he really is.

"Now this is eternal life: that they may know you, the only true God, and Jesus Christ, whom you have sent" (17:3). For this group, the needs of people, not God's will, are first; and what Jesus can do to meet these needs is second. They do not understand the purpose of John's *signs*, and they really don't want to *know* God. Nevertheless, they're always eager for a miracle!

The healing miracles pursued by these people boil down to seeking modern medical cures with a sprinkling of Jesus and, perhaps, faith healers to help them cope. If healing due to medical intervention occurs, Jesus *earns* their applause for a "miracle." If death happens after an eager pursuit of modern medical cures and faith healers for a "miracle," Jesus *merits* their scorn. For these people, Jesus is no different from Asclepius, the Greek god of healing.

Issues, like those mentioned in this book, are not thought about. If the modern medical elites approve organ donation and procurement practices under the Uniform Determination of Death Act (UDDA), then they are not to be questioned. If a treatment exists, then it should be aggressively pursued until death. When it is brought to their attention that medical treatment is not always moral, ethical, or worthy of pursuit, they become indignant and angry.

These emotionally driven hypocrites choose to live in ignorance of the *signs* pointing to Jesus as the Resurrection and the Life. They do not glorify God, nor are the committed to the will of Jesus' heavenly Father. They are eager for healing "miracles" to escape death at all costs because they do not *sincerely* believe in spiritual and eternal life here and now. As Jude says, "They are clouds without rain, blown along by the wind; autumn trees without fruit and up-rooted—twice dead" (v. 12).

However, other people think more deeply, and we see their character traits in the Lazarus account as well. These are often leaders or devoted members of churches. After Jesus raised Lazarus from biological death, John said the episode reached the religious leaders in Jerusalem (11:46–53). A council was assembled to discuss the event comprised of two groups: the Pharisees and Sadducees. The former were pastors at community synagogues, and the latter were priests at the temple.

The Sadducees were the educated elite who were materialists. They craved power, wealth, and prestige in the Roman world. With an air of intellectual hubris, they also denied the supernatural. The Sadducees did not believe in the existence of spirits or in the possibility of miracles and resurrections. At their core, they were anti-supernaturalists.

The people in this group are university dons at seminaries or others attempting to be relevant in the world of academia. For them, Jesus is an opiate for the ignorant and a mythical hope for those in a crisis. According to the elites, heaven, hell, judgment, or a God-breathed spirit animating a human being are not real. Their infallible authority is *Man a Machine*, bolstered by years of rehearsed education, that is motivated by a *passionate zeal* attributed solely to neurochemical by-products emerging from their brains like a mist.

Modern medicine is steeped in philosophical materialism, which simply means our biological brain (organ) is what makes us human. So, to harvest organs from a donor under the UDDA is not murder. They arrive at their conclusions through various philosophical or theological assumptions, some of which we covered throughout the book, especially in chapters three and four.

Unlike the erudite Sadducees, the Pharisees did not deny the supernatural. They believed in spirits, miracles, and resurrections but were self-righteous hypocrites. Many condemned sins in other people, but they did not see themselves as guilty of different types of sins. In practice, they disagreed with the teaching of James: "For whoever keeps the whole law and yet stumbles at just one point is guilty of breaking all of it" (James 2:10). The New Testament has numerous examples of the Pharisaical spirit.

Inconsistent moralism pervades people with this character type. These pastors and devout members at churches rail against abortion, physician-assisted suicide (PAS), and forced organ harvesting in China. They will condemn the woman who gets an abortion after being raped. Then they will honor the woman who chooses to give her life for her unborn baby. A person suffering from cancer choosing suicide is doomed to hell, but one who perseveres in excruciating pain is praised. They call upon God to bring swift judgment on China to root out the evil of forced organ harvesting.

Nevertheless, when Joe needs a heart transplant, they pray to God for an organ donor. Even though they've been instructed about the biological facts mentioned in this book, and the legal fictions facilitating organ harvesting practices in America. They justify the murder of a vulnerable donor by embracing theologians or philosophers they esteem, rather than obey Holy Scripture and cherish the reduced biological life the image-bearer of God possesses.

Of course, none of these character traits are set in stone. We would be in big trouble if they were! Thankfully, there was another group mentioned in John 11. After Lazarus was raised from his biologically dead state, some Jews saw the event and "put their faith" in Jesus as the Resurrection and the Life (v. 45). This group joined the Twelve, Martha, Mary, and Lazarus as committed followers of Jesus.

Every true Christian has a heartfelt commitment to Jesus. He or she says with Peter in John 6, "Lord, to whom shall we go? You have the words of eternal life." *The Christian has a love for the Father that is exclusive, sincere, and seeks to glorify His name by following his revealed will in all circumstances.* A conviction rooted in a fundamental belief that Jesus is the way, the truth, and the life (14:6).

A Few Words in Closing

A Christian cannot be consistent in affirming life begins at conception (at the cellular level) and believe an unresponsive person on life support with a beating heart is dead. This is not a pro-life position, nor is it empirical. Arguing the former life has potential, but the latter does not, passes a judgment about life at odds with the clear teaching of Holy Scripture. The biblical standard for biological death is elapsed time without cardiopulmonary function.

Harvesting organs from donors declared dead under the UDDA is murder in God's eyes, even though it is legal in the United States (US). Further, the foundation for the UDDA is rooted in the Nazi "life unworthy of life" social principles of Beecher, and it is a tool used by the modern organ harvest business in the US to turn a profit. Christians need to oppose the UDDA and these practices.

A bold first step in opposition is refusing to be a registered organ donor. The problem is being *registered* because of the UDDA, not donating organs or tissues, as we noted earlier in the book. Each state has different laws on opting out of being an organ donor, so it's important to look them up. Usually, however, it's just not having the organ donor designation on a driver's license.

A second bold step is speaking out against harvesting organs under the UDDA and the Dead Donor Rule (DDR). These are legal fictions inspired by greed and do not cherish life. They permit a cruel form of active euthanasia, as we noted numerous times in *Harvesting Organs & Cherishing Life*. What we've said in this book needs to be more widely disseminated. Christians need to expose and condemn the UDDA and DDR for what they are, demonic delusions that murder vulnerable image-bearers of God.

Intricately connected with raising our voices against these evils is speaking out against exploitative red markets, black markets, and China's forced harvesting practices. We noted these unscrupulous practices in chapter two. Thankfully, some politicians are raising awareness about these vile practices today. Christians need to unite their voices with these human rights fighters, adding to their message the grace of the Gospel of Jesus Christ.

There is abounding mercy, grace, compassion, and forgiveness in Jesus, even for those in China murdering Uighurs for organs. The same is true for harvest surgeons, anesthesiologists, nurses, and technicians in the United States (US) involved in acts of active euthanasia. This is also true for a person who received an organ transplant from an anonymous donor under the UDDA and for those who made the decision to donate another person's body parts under the same law. These people only need to turn to the

Resurrection and the Life with a sincere and repentant heart, and Jesus says the Creator of life will forgive them.

Then the spirit of life will know the Spirit of life intimately, and one will see by faith the Resurrection and the Life. Then with holy boldness in thought, word, and deed, the Christian will cherish the God of life. Like Dr. Nathanson (the repentant abortion doctor), he or she will condemn the evil of organ harvesting that devalues God-breathed life. As well as Satan's organ procurement puppets and the laws and policies like the UDDA and DDR promoting and empowering them.

More importantly, the Christian with the Holy Spirit of life will look forward with confident expectation for the second coming of the Resurrection and the Life. When complete physical healing will occur, and the *soma psychikon* will become a *soma pneumatikon*. The first resurrection of the healed spirit will blossom into the end-time resurrection of the healed body! On that glorious day, "Death [will be] swallowed up in victory" (1 Cor. 15:54).

Stand fast, Christian, act, and speak! "The God of peace will soon crush Satan under your feet" (Rom. 16:20).